THE POWER

OF

100

TRANSFORMING YOUR LIFE WITH HEALTHY HABITS

DR. JEFFERY ROYAL

Contents

INTRODUCTION

It's easy to disregard our health and well-being in our busy life. We often emphasize job, social commitments, and other duties above self-care. Making time for healthy behaviors, on the other hand, may significantly influence our entire quality of life.

This book is intended to assist you in developing and maintaining 100 healthy habits that may change your life. These habits help you reach your goals and live your best life, whether you want to enhance your physical health, mental well-being, or general happiness.

In the following chapters, we'll look at many elements of health and well-being and provide practical suggestions on how to incorporate good behaviors into your daily routine. This book has something for everyone, from diet and exercise to self-care and stress management.

Before we begin, it is critical to understand that healthy behaviors are not a one-size-fits-all answer. What works for one person may not work for another, so listen to your body and do what feels right. That being said, the habits we'll be covering in this book have been demonstrated to improve the lives of many individuals, and we urge you to give them a go and see how they work for you.

It is also important to note that developing new habits requires time and effort. You won't become a new person overnight, but you may gradually modify your habits and life by making modest, persistent adjustments to your daily routine. Throughout this process, we urge you to be patient and gentle with yourself and appreciate even minor achievements.

So, whether you want to enhance your physical fitness, improve your mental health, or live a more balanced and meaningful life, we hope the habits in this book will inspire and guide you on your path.

THE IMPORTANCE OF HEALTHY HABITS

A healthy lifestyle is vital for general health and longevity. Incorporating healthy habits into your daily routine may aid in preventing chronic illnesses, maintaining a healthy weight, and overall feeling of well-being, both physically and emotionally. In this book, we will look at 100 healthy habits you may use to improve your health and well-being.

Healthy behaviors have several advantages. One of the most important advantages is illness prevention. You may lower your chance of getting chronic illnesses such as heart disease, diabetes, and cancer by eating a balanced diet, exercising frequently, and managing stress. Healthy behaviors may also assist you in maintaining a healthy weight, which is critical for lowering your chance of acquiring obesity-related diseases.

Healthy behaviors have a favorable influence on mental health in addition to physical health. Exercise, for example, has been demonstrated to alleviate melancholy and anxiety symptoms while also improving general mood. A good diet may also enhance mood and cognitive performance, while stress management can improve sleep quality and general mental well-being.

Healthy practices also boost your overall well-being. You may boost your energy levels by including regular exercise, a nutritious diet, and self-care in your daily routine.

Levels increase your sleep quality and boost your overall feeling of well-being. Furthermore, healthy behaviors may help you live a longer, happier life, giving you more time to spend with loved ones and follow your interests.

The advantages of good practices extend beyond personal health. When you put your health and well-being first, you set a good example for people around you and inspire them to do the same. You may also discover that your enhanced energy and mental clarity enable you to be more active and involved in your personal and professional endeavors, which will benefit you and others.

Neglecting healthy behaviors, on the other hand, might have harmful repercussions. Poor diet, inactivity, and persistent stress may all contribute to several health issues. We may feel exhaustion, mood swings, and lower productivity when we ignore our physical and mental health, which may have a severe influence on both our personal and professional lives.

Thankfully, it's never too late to start adopting healthy behaviors into your daily routine. You may enhance your general health and well-being over time by making tiny, incremental adjustments. The 100 healthy habits mentioned in this book are intended to be practical and sustainable, allowing you to adopt them into your life in a comfortable manner.

In the next chapters, we will look at many healthy behaviors relating to diet, exercise, Body and mental health. You can make several adjustments to improve your health and well-being, from eating more whole foods to establishing an exercise program that works for you. You may reap the many advantages of a healthy lifestyle by committing to these healthy habits and incorporating them into your daily routine.

1. SLEEPING ENOUGH EVERY NIGHT

Sleeping well every night is important to maintaining a healthy lifestyle. Sleep is essential for general health and well-being, affecting everything from physical health to cognitive performance and emotional stability. Unfortunately, many individuals fail to get enough sleep because of their hectic schedules, stress, or other circumstances. This section will review the significance of sleep, how to improve your sleeping patterns, and the advantages of obtaining enough sleep each night.

Why Is Sleep So Important?

Sleep is more than simply a way to relax and refresh; it is a vital function that affects practically every area of our health. It is important to get adequate quality sleep each night for:

Physical health: Sleep promotes a healthy immune system, lowers the risk of chronic illness, and promotes physical recovery and development.

Cognitive function: Sleep is necessary for memory consolidation, problem-solving, and decision-making.

Emotional regulation: Getting adequate sleep aids in emotion management and lowers the risk of mood disorders such as sadness and anxiety.

Overall well-being: Getting enough sleep is critical for feeling refreshed, attentive, and ready to face the day.

How Much Sleep Do You Need?

The amount of sleep required varies by age and person, but adults normally need 7-9 hours of quality sleep every night. Children and teens may need more, while elderly individuals may require less. Listening to your body and obtaining adequate sleep every night is important to maintain your overall health and well-being.

Tips for Improving Sleep Habits

There are various things you may take to improve your sleep patterns if you're having trouble getting enough quality sleep each night:

Maintain a regular sleep schedule: Try to go to bed and get up simultaneously every day, including weekends.

Create a bedtime routine: Create a soothing bedtime routine to tell your body it is time to sleep. Examples of such activities include taking a warm bath, reading a book, or practicing relaxation methods such as deep breathing.

Make your bedroom sleep-friendly: To promote sleep, provide a dark, calm, and cold atmosphere. Consider purchasing blackout curtains, a white noise machine, or a plush mattress and pillows.

Avoid stimulating activities before bed: Avoid using electronic gadgets, watching television, or indulging in other stimulating activities before bed since they might make it difficult to fall asleep.

Limit coffee and alcohol: coffee and alcohol may disrupt sleep, so it's best to avoid them, particularly in the hours before bedtime.

The Advantages of Getting Enough Sleep

Getting adequate quality sleep each night provides several health and well-being advantages. Some of the advantages of getting enough sleep are as follows:

- Reduced risk of chronic illnesses such as heart disease, diabetes, and obesity.
- Improved memory and cognitive function.
- Better emotional control and a lower likelihood of mood disorders
- Reduced risk of accidents and injuries related to weariness
- Increased energy and productivity throughout the day

Getting enough sleep each night is critical for leading a healthy, happy, and productive life.

2. DRINKING A LOT OF WATER THROUGHOUT THE DAY

Drinking lots of daily water for general health and well-being is essential. Water is a large body component and essential to numerous physical activities. It regulates body temperature, transports nutrients and oxygen to cells, eliminates waste and toxins, and lubricates joints and tissues.

One of the most important advantages of drinking water is that it keeps us hydrated. Dehydration may cause headaches, dizziness, exhaustion, and constipation, among other symptoms. Our bodies cannot operate properly when dehydrated, which may influence our energy levels and general productivity.

So, how much water should we drink every day? Drinking at least eight 8-ounce glasses of water daily, or roughly 2 liters, is the standard guideline. However, this varies based on age, gender, weight, and activity level. Listening to your body and drinking water whenever you feel thirsty is a smart idea.

Carrying a water bottle with you throughout the day is one strategy to ensure you are drinking enough water. This may be a visual reminder to drink water and simplify staying hydrated, particularly if you are moving or have a hectic schedule. You may also experiment with the setting.

Set a reminder on your phone or computer every hour to take a water break.

Making water more pleasurable is another technique to enhance your water consumption. Infuse your water with fruits, vegetables, or herbs like lemon, cucumber, or mint to enhance taste. This may give your water a pleasant flavor and make drinking more enticing.

Aside from water, it's crucial to be cautious of the other drinks you take during the day. Sugary beverages, such as soda and juice, contain a lot of calories and may lead to weight gain and other health issues. Drinking alcohol may also cause dehydration and other bad health consequences. Therefore, it's crucial to drink moderately and balance alcohol consumption with water consumption.

Drinking enough water throughout the day is a simple yet effective habit that may significantly influence your health and well-being. Staying hydrated may help you have more energy, maintain good digestion, and keep your body running smoothly.

3. EATING A NUTRITIOUS AND BALANCED DIET

One of the most essential things you can do for your health is to eat a balanced and healthy diet. It gives your body the nutrition to perform correctly and stay healthy. A nutritious diet may also assist you in managing your weight, lowering your risk of chronic illnesses, and improving your overall quality of life.

Understanding the fundamentals of nutrition is the first step in eating a nutritious diet. Carbohydrates, proteins, and fats are the three major macronutrients. Carbohydrates are your body's major source of energy, while proteins assist in building and repairing cells and muscles. Fats are required for several processes, including nutrition absorption, hormone production, and brain function.

A balanced plate should have a range of foods from each macronutrient category. Concentrate on whole grains, fruits, and vegetables for carbs. These include fiber, vitamins, minerals, antioxidants, and phytochemicals. Lean meats, fish, eggs, beans, and nuts are good protein sources. Avocado, nuts & seeds, and olive oil are all high in healthy fats.

Regarding food planning and preparation, having a broad notion of what your foods will consist of is beneficial. When you're hungry and pushed for time, this might assist you to avoid making poor decisions. Fill half of your plate with non-starchy veggies, one quarter with protein, and one-quarter with whole grains or other nutritious carbs. This delivers an excellent nutritional balance and may help you feel full and pleased.

It's also vital to keep portion amounts in mind. Even nutritious foods, if consumed in excess, may lead to weight gain. When trying to develop healthy habits, use measuring cups or a food scale to measure your foods.

Another crucial part of healthy eating is including whole foods into your diet. Whole foods are minimally processed and rich in nutrients that promote excellent health. When purchasing, try to choose foods that are as near their natural condition as possible. Fresh fruits and vegetables, nutritious grains like quinoa or brown rice, and less processed meat like chicken or fish may be included.

If you're having trouble incorporating whole foods into your diet, check out different recipes or cooking methods. There are several internet sites for healthy food ideas, and cooking at home may be a fun and creative way to try new foods and tastes.

Finally, don't forget to hydrate and supplement. Water is crucial for overall health because it helps your body maintain optimum pH levels, maintains fluid balance, regulates body temperature, and promotes digestion. Aim for eight glasses of water daily, or more if you're physically active or live in a hot region.

Supplements may also assist to support good nutrition. Consult your doctor or a certified dietitian to see if you are deficient in nutrients that might be addressed with supplements. Remember that supplements should augment, not replace, a balanced diet.

In conclusion, eating a well-balanced and healthy diet is critical for optimum health. Aim for various foods from each macronutrient category, concentrate on whole foods, keep portion sizes in mind, and don't forget about water and supplements. You may enhance your general health and well-being by making tiny adjustments to your diet and developing healthy habits.

4. MAINTAINING A HEALTHY WEIGHT

Maintaining a healthy weight is critical to one's general health and well-being. It may help lower the risk of chronic illnesses, including heart disease, diabetes, and certain malignancies. However, many individuals find achieving and maintaining a healthy weight difficult. Here are some healthy behaviors to help you stay in shape:

Eat a Well-Balanced Diet

Eating a well-balanced diet rich in nutrient-dense foods will help you maintain a healthy weight. Half your food should include fruits and vegetables, a quarter healthy grains, and lean protein sources like chicken, fish, or tofu. Incorporating healthy fats like nuts, seeds, and avocado may also help.

Portion Management

When it comes to maintaining a healthy weight, portion management is essential. Pay attention to serving sizes and use measuring cups and spoons to ensure you eat the right amount. Using smaller dishes might also assist you in eating less.

Avoid processed foods

Processed foods are often heavy in calories, sugar, and bad fats. They may also be deficient in nutrients. Avoiding or restricting processed foods and emphasizing whole, nutrient-dense foods may aid with weight management.

Stay Hydrated

Water consumption is essential for general health, including weight control. Drinking water before foods might make you feel fuller and cause you to eat less. Drink at least eight glasses of water each day.

Limit sugary drinks

Sugary beverages, such as soda, juice, and sports drinks, contain many calories and may lead to weight gain. Sugary beverages should be limited or avoided if you want to maintain a healthy weight.

Mindful Eating

Mindful eating may assist you in maintaining a healthy weight. This includes listening to your hunger and fullness signs, eating carefully, and relishing your food. It also involves avoiding eating distractions, such as television or cell phones.

Exercise regularly

Maintaining a healthy weight requires regular exercise. It may assist you in burning calories, building muscle, and increasing your metabolism. Aim for at least 150 minutes of moderate-intensity activity weekly or 75 minutes of vigorous-intensity exercise.

Strengthening Exercises

When added to your workout program, strength training may help you maintain a healthy weight by increasing lean muscle mass. This may boost your metabolism and help you burn more calories even while you're at rest.

Stay Active Throughout the Day

Staying active throughout the day might also aid with weight management. This includes using the stairs instead of the elevator, parking farther away from your destination, and taking frequent pauses throughout the workday to stand up and stretch.

Get Enough Sleep

Sleep is essential for general health, including weight control. Sleep deprivation may affect hormones that govern hunger and metabolism, resulting in weight gain. Make an effort to obtain seven to nine hours of sleep every night.

By implementing these healthy practices into your lifestyle, you may maintain a healthy weight and lower your risk of chronic illnesses. Start with one or two healthy behaviors and progressively add more as you feel comfortable.

5. EXERCISING REGULARLY

Exercise is an essential component of living a healthy lifestyle. It helps increase physical fitness and maintain a healthy weight and has several mental health advantages, such as stress reduction, mood improvement, and self-confidence boost. Many individuals, however, struggle to make exercise a habit. In this chapter, we will look at the advantages of regular exercise and advise how to include it in your daily routine.

The Advantages of Regular Exercise

Physical health: Regular exercise provides several physical health advantages, including lowering the risk of chronic illnesses such as obesity, type 2 diabetes, and heart disease. It may also help with cardiovascular health, bone density, flexibility, and range of motion.

Mental health: Exercise has been demonstrated to alleviate stress, anxiety, and sadness. Endorphins are substances in the brain that work as natural pain relievers and mood lifters.

Improved Cognitive Function: Studies have indicated that regular exercise improves cognitive function and lowers the risk of cognitive decline in older persons.

Increased Energy: By boosting circulation and oxygen supply to the body, exercise may boost energy levels and minimize weariness.

Better Sleep: Exercise may enhance sleep quality by allowing people to fall asleep sooner and remain asleep longer.

Tips for Exercising Regularly

Choose an Activity You like: Choosing an activity you like and look forward to performing is critical. This will make it simpler for you to adhere to your fitness regimen and incorporate it into your everyday life.

Begin slowly and gradually Increase Intensity: If you're new to exercising, begin with a low-intensity activity like walking or yoga and gradually increase the intensity and length of your exercises.

Set Realistic Goals: Set realistic goals for yourself and celebrate your accomplishments. This will assist you in remaining motivated and devoted to your fitness program.

Find a Workout Partner: Exercising with a friend or family member might help you stay accountable and motivated to keep to your schedule.

Schedule Exercise into Your Day: Treat exercise like any other essential appointment or activity by scheduling it. Incorporate it into your regular regimen. This will make prioritizing and scheduling simpler.

Mix it Up: Use various exercises and activities to keep your workouts interesting and minimize boredom. Cardio, weight training, yoga, and other hobbies such as dancing or martial arts may all be included.

Make Exercise a Priority: Make exercise a priority and an unavoidable part of your everyday routine. This will aid in forming a regular habit and make it simpler to maintain.

Reward Yourself: Celebrate your accomplishments and reward yourself for reaching your goals. This might be as easy as indulging in a favorite dish or soothing bath.

Incorporating regular exercise into your daily routine may offer various physical and mental health advantages. You may build a regular habit and gain the benefits of a healthy lifestyle by picking an activity you love, establishing reasonable goals, and prioritizing exercise.

6. PRACTICE STRESS-REDUCTION TECHNIQUES LIKE MEDITATION OR YOGA

It's not unusual in today's fast-paced world to feel overwhelmed by the demands of everyday living. Stress from a job, relationships, or other commitments may harm our mental and physical health. That's why it's critical to have stress-reduction practices on hand, and two common alternatives are meditation and yoga.

Meditation is a technique that includes concentrating your attention on a certain object, topic, or activity to gain mental clarity and emotional tranquility. Meditation comes in numerous forms, including guided, mindfulness, and transcendental meditation. Regular meditation, regardless of the form, has been demonstrated in studies to decrease stress, anxiety, and depression, as well as increase general well-being.

Finding a quiet space and sitting comfortably with your eyes closed is one method to begin a meditation practice. Concentrate on your breathing and cleanse your mind of any distracting ideas. If your thoughts stray, gently bring them back to your breath. Begin with a few minutes each day and gradually increase to longer sessions.

In contrast, yoga is a physical practice that blends movement, breath, and awareness. There are several styles of yoga, ranging from quiet, restorative yoga to more strenuous vinyasa yoga. Regular yoga practice, like meditation, has been demonstrated in studies to lower stress and anxiety while improving strength, flexibility, and balance.

If you're new to yoga, start with a beginner's class or an online video. Concentrate on good alignment and pay attention to your body's limitations. Remember that yoga is not a competition; it is important to respect your body and practice self-care.

There are numerous additional stress-reduction strategies other than meditation and yoga that you may implement into your life. Among the alternatives are:

Deep breathing exercises: Deep breathing exercises may help soothe the body and lessen stress.

Exercise: It has been established that regular physical exercise reduces stress and improves mood.

Spending time in nature: Spending time in nature may help to relax the body and mind.

Social Support: Connecting with friends and loved ones may help relieve stress and enhance general well-being.

Creative Activities: Painting, writing, or playing music are creative hobbies that may help decrease stress and boost mood.

Finding tactics that work for you and adopting them into your daily routine is the key to successful stress reduction. You may enhance your health and well-being by prioritizing stress reduction.

7. MAINTAINING GOOD HYGIENE, INCLUDING REGULARLY WASHING YOUR HANDS

Good cleanliness is an important element of overall health and fitness. Washing your hands often is one of the most crucial components of hygiene. Hand washing is a simple yet effective activity for preventing the transmission of germs and sickness.

When is it appropriate to wash your hands? Wash your hands in the following scenarios, according to the Centers for Disease Control and Prevention (CDC):

- Before, during, and after food preparation
- Before eating
- Before and after caring for a sick person
- Before and after wound treatment
- After using the restroom
- After you've blown your nose, coughed, or sneezed,
- After coming into contact with an animal, animal feed, or animal waste
- After the disposal of waste

Follow these procedures to wash your hands properly:

- Wet your hands with warm or cold running water.

- Apply soap to your hands and lather them by rubbing them together. Lather your hands' backs, between your fingers, and beneath your nails.
- Rub your hands together for at least 20 seconds. Do you need a timer? Hum the "Happy Birthday" song from beginning to end Twice.
- Rinse your hands thoroughly with clean, running water.
- Dry your hands with a clean towel, or let them air dry.

If you don't have soap or water, you may use an alcohol-based hand sanitizer with at least 60% alcohol. Apply the sanitizer to one hand's palm and massage your hands together until all surfaces of your hands and fingers are dry.

Aside from hand washing, many other crucial hygiene behaviors must be remembered. These are some examples:

- Brushing your teeth twice daily and flossing once daily will help you avoid cavities and gum disease.
- Bathing or showering frequently to keep your skin clean and avoid body odor
- Washing your hair regularly to keep it clean and healthy.
- Keep your nails clean and clipped to avoid the transfer of germs.
- Wearing clean clothing and changing them regularly helps reduce body odor and germ spread.

You can help prevent the spread of sickness and keep yourself and the people around you healthy by practicing excellent hygiene.

8. AVOIDING SMOKING AND EXCESSIVE ALCOHOL CONSUMPTION

Avoiding smoking and excessive alcohol use are two essential practices for good health. These behaviors may have a big influence on your physical and emotional health.

Tobacco use is a substantial risk factor for a wide range of severe health issues, including heart disease, stroke, lung cancer, and respiratory disorders such as chronic bronchitis and emphysema. Furthermore, smoking may cause premature skin aging, teeth loss, and an increased risk of gum disease.

One of the most beneficial things you can do for your health is to stop smoking. It's not simple, but several services are available to assist you with quitting. You may stop smoking by using nicotine replacement treatment, such as gum or patches, or by seeking help from a quit-smoking program or support group. It's important to remember that quitting smoking is a process, and it may take numerous efforts to succeed.

Excessive alcohol drinking may also be harmful to your health. Too much alcohol use may raise your chance of developing liver disease, high blood pressure, heart disease, stroke, and certain forms of cancer. Furthermore, drinking might affect your judgment, leading to accidents or unsafe conduct.

If you want to drink alcohol, you must do so in moderation. Alcohol intake should be limited to no more than one drink per day for women and two drinks per day for males. It's also crucial to take drinking breaks and prevent binge drinking.

It is important to get help if you are having difficulty stopping smoking or reducing your alcohol use. You may get assistance from your doctor, therapist, or a support group.

In addition to the physiological advantages of quitting smoking and drinking less alcohol, these practices may improve your mental health. Both smoking and drinking may be used as coping methods for stress and anxiety, but they can exacerbate these issues in the long term. You may discover better methods to deal with stress and enhance your general well-being by quitting smoking and limiting your alcohol usage.

You are making a commitment to your health and well-being by refraining from smoking and excessive alcohol usage. It is not always easy, but the results are worth the effort. With the correct assistance and tools, you may make these behaviors a permanent part of your healthy lifestyle.

9. FLOSSING AND BRUSHING YOUR TEETH DAILY

Brushing and flossing your teeth may not be the first thing that comes to mind regarding healthy practices. However, excellent dental hygiene is important to overall health and fitness. Gum disease, tooth decay, and even systemic health concerns like heart disease and diabetes may be caused by poor dental hygiene.

Regular brushing and flossing your teeth and gums is essential for good oral health. Brushing your teeth for two minutes twice a day may help eliminate plaque and germs from the surfaces of your teeth. Use fluoride toothpaste and brush in circular strokes, concentrating on each tooth separately. Brush your tongue as well since germs may collect and produce foul breath.

Another key step in maintaining proper dental hygiene is flossing. Flossing aids in the removal of plaque and food particles from between your teeth and along the gumline. If left unchecked, this accumulation may lead to gum disease and tooth decay. To floss correctly:

1. Cut approximately 18 inches of floss and wrap it around your fingers, leaving just a few inches to work with.
2. Using a gentle back-and-forth motion, slide the floss between your teeth.

3. Go under the gumline, but don't snap the floss against your gums.

While brushing and flossing are important for proper dental health, they are not the only considerations. Eating a balanced diet rich in nutrient-dense foods and low in sugar will help keep your teeth and gums healthy. Avoiding tobacco, limiting alcohol use, and keeping hydrated are vital for good dental health.

Regular dental visits are also an important element of maintaining good oral health. You should go to the dentist every six months for a cleaning and checkup. During this time, your dentist may spot any problems with your dental health and address them as needed. They may also advise you on enhancing your oral hygiene regimen and avoiding future problems.

Brushing and flossing daily has additional advantages besides preserving excellent dental health. According to research, regular dental hygiene might enhance cardiovascular health, cognitive function, and even sleep. Brushing and flossing may also help avoid foul breath, boosting your self-esteem and social connections.

Brushing and flossing your teeth regularly may substantially influence your general health and well-being. You may enjoy the advantages of excellent dental health for years to come if you make it a habit.

10. PRACTICING SAFE SEX

Safe sex is an essential component of general health and well-being. Whether you are in a committed relationship or having casual sex, it is important to take precautions to protect yourself and your partner(s) from sexually transmitted diseases (STIs) and unexpected pregnancy.

Using barrier methods of contraception, such as condoms or dental dams, is one of the most effective ways to avoid STIs. These techniques provide a physical barrier between couples, preventing the transmission of infectious body fluids. Condoms are readily accessible and come in various materials and sizes to accommodate personal tastes. They are also effective in preventing unwanted pregnancy; however, using a second method of birth control, such as hormonal contraception, may give further protection.

If you are sexually active, you should also obtain regular STI testing. Many STIs are asymptomatic, which means you may not notice any symptoms even if you are infected. Regular testing may aid in the early detection and treatment of infections, lowering the risk of long-term health consequences and the transmission of the illness to others.

In addition to barrier techniques and testing, open and honest communication with sexual partners is essential for practicing safe sex. This includes addressing sexual history, STI status, and other issues.

Before engaging in sexual activity, utilize contraception. It may be a tough talk to have, but it is essential for maintaining excellent sexual health and minimizing illness transmission.

Respecting your own and your partner's limits is also part of practicing safe sex. Consent is a fundamental component of good sexual interactions, and all people involved should freely grant it. It is critical to have open and continuing discussions about boundaries and consent and be prepared to respect and alter them as required.

Finally, it's important to understand that practicing safe sex is about more than simply avoiding bad outcomes; it's also about creating happy sexual encounters. You and your partner(s) may experience sexual intimacy in a manner that improves your overall physical and mental well-being when you and your partner(s) feel secure, comfortable, and appreciated.

Finally, practicing safe sex is an important element of general health and well-being. This includes utilizing barrier contraception, receiving STI testing regularly, speaking honestly with sexual partners, respecting boundaries and consent, and emphasizing the significance of happy sexual encounters. Adopting these precautions protects yourself and your partner(s) against harmful health effects.

11. VISITING YOUR DOCTOR REGULARLY FOR CHECK-UPS AND SCREENINGS

Regular medical check-ups and tests are critical to preserving your health and well-being. These visits allow one to discover possible health issues before they become significant problems, obtain advice, and help maintain healthy behaviors.

Your age, gender, family history, and other personal characteristics will determine the frequency and kind of tests advised. Your doctor may prescribe the following screenings:

Blood Pressure: High blood pressure, often known as hypertension, is a significant risk factor for heart disease and stroke. Blood pressure checks are suggested for all individuals, and those with high blood pressure or other risk factors may need to be done more regularly.

Cholesterol: High cholesterol levels may also put you at risk for heart disease and stroke. If you have a family history of high cholesterol or heart disease or additional risk factors such as obesity or diabetes, your doctor may prescribe cholesterol screening.

Diabetes: Diabetes is a disorder in which your body's ability to manage blood sugar levels is impaired. It may lead to a variety of dangerous problems if left untreated. Your doctor may prescribe diabetes screening if you have risk factors for diabetes, such as obesity, high blood pressure, or a family history of diabetes.

Cancer: Depending on your age and gender, your doctor may prescribe mammograms, colonoscopies, or prostate examinations.

Vision and hearing: Your vision and hearing may decline as you age. Regular screenings may aid in the early detection of problems and the prevention of future deterioration.

In addition to these checks, your doctor may advise you to be vaccinated against infectious illnesses, such as the flu shot or the COVID-19 vaccine.

Even if you feel well, scheduling frequent check-ups with your doctor is important. These appointments allow you to address any problems you may have and get advice and support for maintaining healthy behaviors. Your doctor may also assist you in managing chronic diseases such as diabetes or high blood pressure and can refer you to specialists or other healthcare professionals as required.

In addition to seeing your doctor regularly, there are activities you may do to maintain your health in between consultations. These are some examples:

Keeping track of your symptoms: Note any changes in your health or new symptoms and discuss them with your doctor at your next visit.

Monitoring your vital signs: Using a blood pressure cuff or other monitoring equipment, you may check your blood pressure, heart rate, and other vital signs at home.

Keeping track of your medications: Make a note of all the medicines you're taking, including OTCs and vitamins, and discuss it with your doctor at each visit.

Maintaining a healthy lifestyle: Maintaining good health requires eating a balanced diet, keeping physically active, getting adequate sleep, and managing stress.

By being proactive about your health and collaborating with your doctor, you may help avoid and manage many common health issues and live a long and healthy life.

12. GETTING VACCINATIONS AS NEEDED

Vaccinations are one of the most effective methods to keep infectious diseases at bay. Vaccines expose the immune system to a weakened or dead version of a virus or bacterium, stimulating antibody production. If the individual is exposed to the virus or bacterium again, the antibodies will detect and fight it. Vaccinations have eliminated illnesses such as smallpox and significantly reduced the prevalence of others, such as measles and polio.

They not only protect those who get immunizations, but they also contribute to herd immunity. Herd immunity occurs when a significant enough proportion of the population is immunized, making it harder for the illness to spread even among people who are not immunized, such as those who are unable to obtain vaccinations for medical reasons. Herd immunity protects vulnerable people such as babies, the elderly, and those with compromised immune systems who are more prone to the consequences of infectious illness.

Several vaccinations are available, and the recommended immunization schedule differs depending on age, health condition, work, and other variables. The Centers for Disease Control and Prevention (CDC) publishes immunization schedule instructions for children and adults on their website.

Measles, mumps, rubella (MMR), polio, hepatitis B, and varicella (chickenpox) immunizations are common for youngsters. Adults may get influenza, tetanus, diphtheria, pertussis (Tdap), shingles, and pneumonia vaccines.

It is crucial to recognize that immunizations can have dangers, albeit major adverse effects are uncommon. Some persons may have mild adverse effects such as pain or edema at the injection site, fever, or headache. Any concerns regarding immunizations should be discussed with a healthcare professional, and any adverse reactions should be reported to the Vaccine Adverse Event Reporting System (VAERS).

Some people may be unable to get vaccinations due to medical conditions such as allergies or weakened immune systems. These people must depend on herd immunity to protect themselves from infectious illnesses.

Vaccinations and their safety have been the subject of debate in recent years. Some people are afraid to obtain vaccinations because they are concerned about possible adverse effects or believe that vaccines are ineffective. However, the vast bulk of scientific evidence supports vaccination safety and efficacy.

It is critical to seek out reputable vaccination information sources and be wary of misinformation transmitted via social media or other channels. Healthcare providers and public health organizations such as the CDC are reliable sources of information on vaccinations.

Finally, immunizations are important to public health and individual well-being. They have played an important role in preventing the spread of infectious illnesses and safeguarding vulnerable people. It is important to adhere to prescribed immunization schedules and to consult with a healthcare physician if you have any concerns.

13. LIMITING SCREEN TIME, ESPECIALLY BEFORE BED

Many of us spend a substantial amount of time in front of screens in today's digital world, whether for business, enjoyment, or communication. While technology has many benefits, it also has significant negatives, especially regarding our sleep and general health.

Blue light produced by electronic gadgets such as phones, tablets, and laptops may disrupt our circadian cycle and inhibit melatonin synthesis, a hormone that governs sleep. This may make falling and staying asleep more difficult, resulting in exhaustion, mood problems, and other undesirable consequences.

Excessive screen time has been linked to a variety of health concerns, including eye strain, migraines, neck and back discomfort, and even obesity. It may also harm our mental health since social media and other online activities can exacerbate feelings of isolation, anxiety, and sadness.

To counteract these harmful impacts, we must restrict our screen usage, particularly in the hours preceding up to sleep. Experts advise avoiding screens for at least an hour before bed and instead indulging in soothing activities like reading, bathing, or doing mindfulness exercises.

You may take additional actions, in addition to avoiding devices before bed, to minimize your total screen usage and encourage better behaviors. Setting limits on your daily use is one option. You may do this by utilizing applications or features that measure and limit your screen time or simply by deliberately taking breaks and participating in other activities throughout the day.

Another method is to reconsider your relationship with technology and examine how you may use it more intentionally and in a more balanced manner. Setting limits around work-related activities, emphasizing face-to-face contacts over digital ones, or finding other sources of amusement that do not require screens are all examples of this.

Finally, being conscious and purposeful about how we use technology in our everyday lives is the key to minimizing screen time and developing better behaviors. We can develop a better and more balanced relationship with screens and technology and enhance our general health and well-being by making little adjustments and remaining dedicated to our goals.

14. IF YOU WORK AT A DESK JOB, TAKE BREAKS AND STRETCH

If you work at a desk job, you probably spend a lot of time sitting each day. While sitting at a desk may seem innocuous, extended sitting may harm your health. Sedentism has been related to an increased risk of obesity, heart disease, and other health issues. To offset the detrimental consequences of sitting, taking breaks and stretching often during the day is essential.

Taking breaks during the workday might help you spend less time sitting down. Even little pauses, like getting up to refill your water bottle or heading to the restroom, might be useful. Try to take a couple of longer breaks during the day to exercise your body and get some fresh air if possible. You may stroll outdoors, stretch lightly, or just get up and move about for a few minutes.

Stretching and taking breaks may increase flexibility, decrease muscular tension, and avoid injury. Here are some stretches to perform at your desk:

Neck Stretches: Tilt your head slowly to one side, bringing your ear near your shoulder. Hold for a few seconds before repeating on the other side. You may also stretch front and backward by gradually lowering your chin to your chest and then gaze up towards the ceiling.

Shoulder Rolls: In a circular motion, roll your shoulders forward and backward. This might help you relax your upper back and neck.

Wrist and forearm stretches: Extend one arm out in front of you, with your palm facing down. Gently draw your fingers towards your body with your other hand until you feel a stretch in your wrist and forearm. Hold for a few seconds before repeating on the other side.

Seated Spinal Twist: Sit on your chair sideways with your feet flat on the floor. Slowly rotate to the right, looking over your shoulder, with your left hand on the outside of your right knee. Hold for a few seconds before repeating on the other side.

Hamstring Stretch: Stretch your hamstrings by sitting on the edge of your chair with your feet flat on the floor. Extend one leg before you, with your heel on the floor, and your toes pointing up. Lean forward from your hips till the back of your thigh stretches. Hold for a few seconds before repeating on the other side.

Remember to take slow breaths when stretching and to never overextend yourself. Stop immediately if you experience any pain or discomfort.

Incorporating exercise and stretching into your work may offer several health and well-being advantages. You may enhance your flexibility, decrease muscular stress, and increase productivity and attention by taking frequent pauses and stretching. So, the next time you sit at your desk for a lengthy amount of time, stretch. Your mind and body will be grateful.

Walking is a simple yet effective type of exercise with several health advantages. It is a low-impact workout that can be done anywhere with no specific equipment or gym membership required. Walking regularly may help you maintain a healthy weight, lower your risk of chronic illnesses, and enhance your physical and mental health.

Adults should strive for at least 150 minutes of moderate-intensity aerobic activity each week, according to the Centers for Disease Control and Prevention (CDC). Walking 3-4 kilometers per hour fast may satisfy this requirement and give considerable health benefits. Here are some ways that frequent walking might improve your life:

Weight Management:
Walking is an efficient technique to maintain a healthy weight or reduce weight if done regularly. Depending on weight and activity, a 30-minute brisk walk may burn between 150 and 200 calories. These calories might pile up over time and result in weight reduction. Walking also helps to develop lean muscle mass, which may boost metabolism and help you burn calories even when you're not moving.

Reduced Risk of Chronic Diseases:
Walking may help lower the risk of chronic illnesses such as heart disease, diabetes, and stroke. Walking daily may help decrease blood pressure and enhance blood circulation,

improve blood sugar levels, as is inflammation in the body. These characteristics may help reduce the risk of chronic illnesses and improve general health.

Increased Mental Health: Walking has been demonstrated to improve mental health. Walking regularly may help to alleviate stress, anxiety, and sadness. Walking also causes the production of endorphins, which are the body's natural feel-good chemicals. Walking outside in nature may also have a relaxing impact and enhance mood.

Increased Energy and Stamina: Walking regularly will help you gain energy and stamina. Walking increases circulation and oxygen flow to the body, which boosts energy levels. Walking also improves the cardiovascular system, allowing you to do everyday tasks more comfortably and less wearily.

Better Sleep: Walking may help enhance the quality and length of your sleep. Walking is an excellent exercise for individuals of all ages and fitness levels since it has been proven to help sleep in general. Walking may help lower tension and anxiety, which can disrupt sleep. Morning and afternoon walks may also assist in regulating the body's natural sleep-wake cycle.

Walking, in general, is a simple and efficient approach to enhance both your physical and emotional health. It is a simple practice to integrate into your routine, regardless of

It may be a quick stroll at lunch or a longer walk in the evening. Wear comfortable shoes and clothes, and begin gently, gradually increasing intensity and time. Walking daily may revolutionize your life and enhance your overall health and well-being.

16. MAINTAINING A POSITIVE OUTLOOK AND ATTITUDE

Maintaining a positive outlook and attitude is critical to general health and well-being. How we think and feel greatly influences our physical health, mental health, and overall quality of life. According to research, individuals with a positive view and attitude tend to live longer, healthier lives and are better suited to deal with stress and hardship.

Improved mental health is a fundamental advantage of a happy mindset. An optimistic mindset may help minimize sadness, anxiety, and stress symptoms. Positive thinking has been related to higher serotonin levels and other neurotransmitters connected to better mood and lower stress. Individuals who are cheerful are also more resilient and better equipped to deal with difficult situations.

Keeping a good attitude may also have considerable physical health advantages. According to research, those who retain a happy attitude are less likely to acquire chronic illnesses such as heart disease, stroke, and diabetes. Furthermore, a cheerful attitude has been linked to increased immunological function, lower blood pressure, and less inflammation.

So, how can we keep a happy attitude and outlook? One method is to practice thankfulness. Gratitude entails concentrating on the good parts of our life and appreciating what we have. Gratitude practice has been demonstrated in studies to boost mood, decrease stress, and promote emotions of well-being. Keeping a gratitude book, expressing appreciation to others, and taking time to appreciate life's wonderful things are easy methods to practice thankfulness.

Another strategy to keep a happy attitude is to surround oneself with positive people. According to research, Individuals with good social ties are happier and healthier than those who are socially isolated. Emotional support, encouragement, and a feeling of belonging may all be provided by positive social ties. Surrounding yourself with positive individuals may also help us retain a good attitude when facing difficulties or hardship.

Finally, we must take care of ourselves physically and psychologically. Self-care is making time for things that benefit our health, such as exercise, relaxation, and hobbies we like. By emphasizing self-care, we can better deal with stress and retain a positive mindset.

Finally, having a good outlook and attitude is critical for general health and well-being. A good attitude may help enhance one's mental, physical, and overall quality of life. We may keep a positive mindset and live happier, healthier lives by practicing appreciation, surrounding ourselves with good people, and emphasizing self-care.

17. SETTING ACHIEVABLE GOALS AND WORKING TOWARD THEM

Setting and working toward achievable goals is critical to developing healthy behaviors. It might be difficult to keep motivated and focused on the changes we want if we don't have goals. On the other hand, setting unreasonable or unreachable goals might lead to dissatisfaction and a feeling of failure. It's important to balance challenging ourselves and creating attainable goals.

Setting goals requires being detailed and clear about what you want to accomplish. It might be tough to discern whether you're making progress if your goals are vague or generic. For example, what does that entail if you want to "eat healthier"? Instead, aim to "eat at least three servings of vegetables every day" or "cook dinner at home at least four times a week."

Goals should not only be defined but also quantifiable. This implies you should be able to monitor your progress and determine how far you've come. Measurable goals enable you to appreciate little accomplishments while remaining inspired to continue. For example, if you want to run a 5K, you may measure your progress by jogging lesser distances and progressively increasing your mileage weekly.

Another important part of goal-setting is making them attainable. While it is necessary to push oneself, choosing goals that are too demanding or unreasonable might lead to failure. When defining goals, keep your present talents and resources in mind. For example, if you've never jogged before, setting a goal of running a marathon in six months may be unrealistic. Begin with a lesser goal, such as running a 5K or jogging for 30 minutes without stopping.

Setting goals relevant to your health and well-being is also vital. When making goals, keep your principles and priorities in mind. For example, if you value spending time with your family, you might make a goal to go for a daily walk with your wife or children. Setting a goal to practice yoga or meditation regularly may be beneficial if you suffer from stress and worry.

Finally, goals should be time-bound. Setting a precise timeline for reaching your objective is one example of this. A deadline instills a feeling of urgency and drives you to act. It's easy to postpone and put off making adjustments when there's no deadline. For example, if you want to lose 10 pounds, give yourself three months to attain that goal.

Monitoring your progress and making modifications as required while working toward your goals is critical. Checking your progress regularly might help you stay motivated and on track. If you're not progressing toward your goal, it may be time to rethink your strategy and modify it as required. For example, if you cannot cook supper at home four times per week as planned, consider reducing your aim to three times per week or experimenting with food prep to simplify it.

Finally, choosing attainable goals is an important element of developing healthy behaviors. Be specific, measurable, achievable, relevant, and time-bound while making goals.

Target your progress regularly and make modifications as required to keep on target. You may develop healthy habits that will last a lifetime if you have the appropriate mentality and approach.

18. ENGAGING IN SELF-CARE ACTIVITIES SUCH AS BATHING OR GETTING A MASSAGE

Self-care is important to sustaining one's physical, emotional, and mental well-being. Self-care activities may help you decrease stress, enhance sleep quality, and relax. Taking a bath and having a massage are two common self-care activities that many people enjoy. In this part, we'll look at the advantages of these activities and give you some pointers on how to include them in your self-care regimen.

Bathing is a simple but powerful form of self-care that can be readily included in your everyday routine. A warm bath may aid in the relaxation of muscles, the reduction of tension, and the promotion of emotions of peace and tranquility. Adding Epsom salt to your bathwater might boost these advantages even further. Epsom salt is high in magnesium, a mineral that aids in reducing inflammation, improving muscle and nerve function, and promoting relaxation.

To take a bath for self-care, first, create a calm setting. Dim the lights, light a few candles, and put on some soothing music. Fill the tub halfway with warm water and sprinkle with a cup or two of Epsom salt. Soak for at least 20 minutes in the bath, taking slow breaths and letting yourself relax. Aromatherapy advantages may also be obtained by adding essential oils to your bathwater. Lavender oil, for example, is recognized for its relaxing characteristics and may aid in anxiety reduction and relaxation.

Getting a massage is another popular self-care activity. Massage therapy is the manipulation of soft tissues in the body to promote relaxation, pain relief, and general well-being. Massage treatment may aid in reducing muscular tension and discomfort, as well as improving circulation and the immune system.

Consider reserving a session with a professional massage therapist to include massage into your self-care regimen. They may tailor the massage to your unique requirements and tastes. You may also attempt self-massage methods at home with a foam roller or massage ball. These instruments may aid in the release of muscular tension and the promotion of relaxation. You may also use essential oils to increase the advantages of massage. Peppermint oil, for example, is well-known for its cooling and energizing properties, and it may aid in the relief of muscular aches and stress.

Aside from taking a bath and having a massage, you might attempt several additional self-care activities. Some suggestions include doing yoga or meditation, taking a natural stroll, reading a book, or napping. Finding things that you like and that make you feel rested and energized is the key.

It is important to prioritize self-care in your everyday routine. Taking care of oneself helps not just you but also everyone around you. When calm, relaxed, and invigorated, you can better deal with stress and obstacles in your everyday life.

Finally, having a bath and getting a massage are two beneficial self-care activities that may aid in relaxation, stress reduction, and general well-being. Whether you go to a massage therapist or take a soothing bath at home, the important thing is to make self-care a regular part of your routine. You'll be better able to face life's difficulties with renewed energy and vigor if you care for yourself.

19. SPENDING TIME IN NATURE

It has been shown that spending time in nature offers various physical and mental health advantages. In today's fast-paced world, it's easy to get engrossed in the hustle and bustle of daily living, which may lead to feelings of stress, worry, and burnout. On the other hand, taking time to immerse yourself in nature may bring much-needed relief from the daily grind and boost your general well-being.

Studies have proven that spending time in nature improves mental wellness. According to research published in the Journal of Environmental Psychology, spending only 20 minutes in a natural environment, such as a park or forest, may substantially drop cortisol, a stress hormone. Furthermore, spending time in nature has been related to better mood, enhanced feelings of relaxation, and reduced sadness and anxiety symptoms.

Spending time in nature may offer physical health advantages in addition to mental health benefits. Spending time in green areas was linked to a decreased chance of acquiring chronic illnesses such as cardiovascular disease and diabetes, according to one research published in the International Journal of Environmental Health Research. Furthermore, time spent in nature has been demonstrated to enhance sleep quality, decrease inflammation in the body, and increase the immune system.

So, how can you include more natural elements into your everyday routine? There are methods to connect with nature, even in a city or urban setting. A stroll in a park or nature reserve, a hike, or just sitting outdoors with a cup of tea may all give the advantages of spending time in nature. Incorporating plants and natural features into your living area may also assist in bringing nature inside.

It's worth noting that spending time in nature does not have to be a solo pastime. Connecting with people in nature might have even more advantages. Joining a hiking club, taking outdoor yoga or fitness courses, or just going for a stroll with a buddy may give social connection and advantages of being in nature.

Including nature in your daily life may be a simple but effective method to enhance your overall health and well-being. Making time for nature, whether it's spending a few minutes sitting outdoors and soaking up the sun, going on a weekend trek, or finding ways to bring the natural world inside, may positively influence your mental and physical health.

20. BUILDING AND MAINTAINING SUPPORTIVE RELATIONSHIPS WITH FAMILY AND FRIENDS

Building and maintaining supportive relationships with family and friends is critical for general health and well-being. Positive connections with family and friends may give emotional support, aid in stress management, and even enhance physical health results. Poor connections with family and friends, on the other hand, may have a detrimental impact on both mental and physical health. In this part, we'll discuss the significance of supporting relationships and provide suggestions for developing and sustaining good relationships with people closest to us.

According to research, social support has been related to various health advantages, including better mental health outcomes, decreased rates of chronic illness, and even enhanced lifespan. According to one research, social support is connected with a lower risk of death, with those who reported strong social ties having a 50% higher probability of surviving than those who reported fewer relationships. Other research has connected social support to reduced stress hormone levels, greater immune system function, and better cardiovascular health.

So, how can we cultivate and sustain supportive connections with family and friends? Communication is an important component. Good communication is required for healthy relationships, and it entails both listening and efficiently expressing oneself in good interactions. Being an active listener is critical, which involves paying attention to what the other person is saying rather than just waiting your time to speak. It is also crucial to express oneself openly and honestly while being respectful of the sentiments and ideas of others.

Spending quality time together is also crucial. This does not necessarily imply spending much time together but making that time meaningful and joyful. This may be as easy as a phone conversation or video chat with a loved one who lives far away or as complex as organizing a fun activity, such as walking or trying a new restaurant.

Trust, respect, and reciprocal support are also components of supportive partnerships. This includes being there during tough times, enjoying one another's triumphs, and offering emotional support when necessary. It is important to be honest and trustworthy and treat one another with love and understanding.

Building and sustaining helpful connections is not always simple. Conflicts may emerge when family and friends have opposing viewpoints, ideas, and attitudes. When this occurs, it is critical to approach the problem with an open mind, actively listen to the other person's point of view, and attempt to establish common ground. It is also critical to establish and clearly explain limits so that everyone involved understands what is and is not acceptable.

Finally, developing and sustaining supportive connections with family and friends is critical to general health and well-being. Positive connections provide emotional support, enhance mental and physical health results, and even extend one's life. Communicating effectively, spending quality time together, and giving mutual support and respect to create and sustain good relationships are critical. While disagreements are inevitable, addressing them with an open mind and transparent communication may help to resolve them and enhance relationships in the long term.

21. DOING ACTIVITIES THAT BRINGS YOU JOY AND HAPPINESS

In today's fast-paced world, it's easy to get engrossed in the minutiae of daily life and forget to make time for the things that bring us pleasure and satisfaction. Engaging in things that offer us pleasure, whether spending time with loved ones, following a creative interest, or just appreciating the beauty of nature, is a crucial element of living a healthy and meaningful life.

According to research, participating in joyful activities might improve our general well-being. For example, research published in the Journal of Good Psychology found that those who participated in more frequent, diverse, enjoyable activities reported greater life satisfaction and good feelings. Another research published in the Journal of Happiness Studies discovered that participating in joyful activities helped alleviate sadness and anxiety symptoms.

Despite the advantages of participating in joyful hobbies, many of us may struggle to prioritize these activities in our busy lives. We may feel guilty about taking time for ourselves or believe we should focus on more "productive" duties instead.

To overcome these obstacles, we may change our thinking and see joyful activities as an essential element of self-care. Similarly, we prioritize exercise and a nutritious diet We should emphasize activities that promote our mental and emotional well-being and those that promote our physical health.

Making a list of things that offer you pleasure and committing to doing at least one of these activities each day is one method to integrate more joyful activities into your life. This might involve anything from taking a nature walk, making a wonderful dinner, or engaging in a creative activity.

It might also be beneficial to arrange time for these activities in your calendar to ensure that you do them daily. This might help you remain responsible and include enjoyable things in your daily routine.

Remembering that having fun doesn't have to be a solitary affair is vital. On the other hand, engaging in things that offer you delight alongside loved ones might be an even more potent method to improve your well-being. Sharing delightful experiences with people may assist in building relationships and boost emotions of pleasure and satisfaction, whether taking a dancing class with your spouse or going on a walk with friends.

Finally, participating in joyful activities is essential to leading a healthy and meaningful life. We may minimize stress, raise our mood, and improve our general well-being by prioritizing things that offer us pleasure and happiness.

22. LISTENING TO MUSIC THAT MAKES YOU HAPPY

Music has been a vital aspect of human civilization for thousands of years. It can elicit deep emotions, memories, and even bodily reactions in people. A recent study has revealed that listening to music may have various health advantages, including stress reduction, mood enhancement, and relaxation.

When it comes to health, one of the most significant components in sustaining general well-being is stress reduction. Chronic stress has been related to a variety of health issues, including hypertension, cardiovascular disease, and depression. Music has been demonstrated to be an excellent stress-reduction strategy, slowing the heart rate, lowering blood pressure, and lowering levels of the stress hormone cortisol.

Music has been shown to increase mood, induce relaxation, and lower stress. According to research published in the Journal of Positive Psychology, individuals who listened to uplifting music had higher happiness and positive affect levels. Similarly, according to research published in the Journal of Music Therapy, listening to calming music might reduce anxiety and increase relaxation.

However, it is not just the style of music that is important; the personal connection to the song may also play a role. It plays a key part in its health benefits. According to research published in the Journal of Advanced Nursing, patients who listened to music they liked had lower pain levels and higher sentiments of well-being. This shows that the emotional connection to music might increase its health benefits.

Listening to music may have physical advantages in addition to psychological ones. Music has been found in studies to improve endurance and performance during exercise by distracting from sensations of weariness and promoting a happy attitude. Participants in a research published in the Journal of Sports Medicine and Physical Fitness who listened to music while cycling had better endurance and performance than those who rode silently.

While listening to music has several health advantages, it is crucial to recognize that not all music is made equal. The sort of music that aids relaxation and stress reduction varies depending on personal choice and individual experiences. Some people believe that classical music aids relaxation, but others prefer more current music genres such as jazz or ambient music. Furthermore, the loudness and pace of the music might influence its efficiency in encouraging relaxation and stress reduction.

Finally, listening to music that makes you happy may have various health advantages, including stress reduction, mood enhancement, and relaxation. A personal connection to music may also be important in its health advantages.

It may heighten the emotional reaction to the music. When adding music to a wellness regimen, it's crucial to look for music that promotes relaxation and stress reduction and matches your unique interests and experiences. Individuals may gain music's physical, psychological, and emotional advantages by integrating it into their everyday lives.

23. LAUGHING REGULARLY

Laughter has been proven to have various mental and physical health advantages. Laughter not only brings pleasure and happiness but is also a natural stress reliever, increases social bonds, and improves general health.

Endorphins, the body's natural feel-good chemicals, are released when we laugh. Endorphins are responsible for pain relief and sensations of pleasure and contentment. This natural endorphin release may help alleviate stress and anxiety, resulting in an overall improvement in mental health.

Laughter has also been found to improve physical wellness. A big belly laugh may help strengthen the immune system, improve blood flow and oxygenation throughout the body, and even provide natural exercise for the diaphragm and abdominal muscles. Laughing may also help decrease blood pressure and minimize the risk of heart disease.

Laughter may be a terrific way to connect with people and improve social ties. Shared laughing helps individuals connect and may even help alleviate uncomfortable circumstances. We experience a feeling of connection and community when we laugh with others, which may be particularly essential during times of stress or loneliness.

So, how can we add more humor to our lives? One method is to look for comedy in ordinary situations. Finding ways to laugh every day, whether by watching a hilarious movie or TV program, reading a humorous book or comic, or just exchanging jokes with friends and family, may significantly influence our general health and well-being.

It's also crucial to keep in mind that laughing spreads. We encourage people to laugh when we laugh with them, generating a positive feedback loop that may lead to even more laughter and delight. So, the next time you're anxious or depressed, try to find something to chuckle about - you may be amazed at how much better you feel!

Finally, laughing is a sometimes ignored part of general health and well-being. Including more laughing in our lives may have several mental and physical health advantages, such as less stress and anxiety, enhanced physical health, and stronger social ties. So, go ahead and chuckle at anything today - your body and mind will reward you.

24. KEEPING A GRATITUDE JOURNAL AND FOCUSING ON THE POSITIVE ASPECTS OF YOUR LIFE

Practicing thankfulness is one of the most effective practices for increasing your overall well-being. Gratitude is the act of being grateful and appreciative of the good things in one's life, no matter how little they may seem. You may enhance your mood, decrease stress, and promote emotions of pleasure and satisfaction by concentrating on the positive.

Keeping a gratitude notebook is an excellent technique to promote thankfulness. This entails spending a few minutes each day writing down things you are thankful for. These might be large or tiny and range from having a supportive buddy to savoring a hot cup of coffee in the morning.

Keeping a thankfulness notebook has been demonstrated in studies to have a substantial influence on your general well-being. One research participant who maintained a thankfulness notebook for three weeks reported feeling more positive, content with their lives, and connected to others. They also reported fewer bodily symptoms like headaches and stomachaches and improved sleep.

One of the reasons gratitude writing works so well is because it transforms your perspective from negative to positive. Our brains are often designed to concentrate on unpleasant parts of our lives, such as challenges and pressures. You may rewire your brain to recognize the good in your life by purposefully concentrating on the positive, which can lead to increased emotions of happiness and well-being.

Another advantage of thankfulness writing is that it might assist you in dealing with challenging circumstances. When we confront difficulties or failures, it is easy to get mired in negative feelings such as irritation or disappointment. We may adjust our viewpoint and discover hope and optimism even in tough circumstances by concentrating on the positive aspects of our lives.

To begin a gratitude notebook, set out a few minutes each day to focus on what you are thankful for. Make at least three notes, and be as descriptive as possible. Instead of saying, "I'm grateful for my family," you may say, "I'm grateful for my sister's sense of humor and how she always makes me laugh."

You might also try utilizing prompts to get started. Some common prompts are:

- What brought a grin to my face today?
- What do I like about my relationships?
- What aspects of my job or profession make me grateful?
- What am I grateful for in terms of my physical health?
- What do I like about my house or living situation?

Remember that regularity is the key to gratitude writing. Even if you just have a few minutes, try to make it a regular habit.

You may notice that your viewpoint evolves, and you begin to perceive more and more of the wonderful in your life.

There are additional strategies to promote thankfulness in your everyday life besides gratitude blogging. These might include:

- Thanking individuals for their compassion or support
- Observing and enjoying the beauty around you, such as a lovely sunset or a blooming flower
- Taking time to appreciate and enjoy small pleasures, such as a good dinner or a warm hug
- Mindfulness practice and being present in the moment
- Volunteering or contributing to charity to assist people in need

Incorporating these activities into your daily routine will assist you in cultivating a more positive and thankful mentality, which can have far-reaching effects on your entire well-being.

25. MINDFULNESS PRACTICE AND BEING PRESENT IN THE MOMENT

Mindfulness and being present in the moment are critical components of general well-being. The practice of devoting one's attention to the present moment without judgment is known as mindfulness. This technique has been demonstrated to boost mood, decrease stress and anxiety, increase concentration and attention, and even improve physical health.

Mindfulness may be practiced in various methods, including meditation, yoga, breathing exercises, and body scan techniques. Focusing on the breath is one of the easiest and most effective techniques to cultivate mindfulness. This can be done anywhere, at any time, and may be useful for lowering tension and anxiety.

To begin, sit on a chair or the floor comfortably. Close your eyes or lower your gaze and focus on your breathing. Take note of how your breath moves in and out of your body. You may feel the movement of your breath by placing your palm on your tummy or chest.

Thoughts may occur while you concentrate on your breathing. This is both natural and to be anticipated. When your mind wanders, just return your focus to the breath without judgment or criticism. You may find it useful to see your ideas as passing clouds. Allow them to fade away while you focus on your breathing.

This kind of mindfulness practice may assist in relieving stress and anxiety by focusing on the current moment rather than thinking about the past or the future. It may also boost your mood by allowing you to focus on the present moment and enjoy the little things in life.

Aside from mindfulness meditation, several more methods exist to develop awareness in everyday life. Take a few deep breaths before commencing a task, such as checking email or starting a meeting, as a basic technique. This might help you concentrate and center your attention.

Engaging in tasks that need your whole concentration, such as cooking, gardening, or playing an instrument, is another method to develop mindfulness. These exercises might help you focus on the present moment and produce emotions of peace and relaxation.

Mindfulness practice may also offer physical health advantages. Studies have found mindfulness to help relieve chronic pain, regulate blood pressure, and enhance sleep quality.

In conclusion, practicing mindfulness and being present in the moment may be a powerful strategy for enhancing general well-being. This technique may help you decrease tension and worry, boost your mood, increase focus and attention, and even boost physical health. There are several methods to cultivate mindfulness, ranging from meditation to participating in activities that need your undivided attention. By incorporating mindfulness into your everyday routine, you may reap the benefits of this powerful discipline.

26. ESTABLISHING BOUNDARIES AND SAYING NO WHEN NEEDED

Humans often feel obligated to satisfy others, which may lead to overcommitment and disregarding our needs. On the other hand, learning to establish boundaries and say no when required is a crucial part of preserving our general health and well-being.

If we fail to establish limits, we may develop tension, exhaustion, and even hatred towards others we believe are taking advantage of us. On the other hand, setting limits helps us take charge of our lives and prioritize our own needs, leading to greater satisfaction and contentment.

Identifying our wants and priorities is an important step in creating limits. This is pausing to consider what is essential to us and what we must do to preserve our physical, emotional, and mental health. We may begin to convey our requirements to others clearly and aggressively if we clearly grasp them.

It is important to understand that creating limits does not imply being selfish or indifferent about others. Instead, it entails striking a balance between our wants and the needs of others. This may include limiting the amount of time and energy we dedicate to specific hobbies or relationships and learning to say no when necessary.

Learning to say no might be especially difficult for those who strongly desire to please others. However, it is important to remember that saying no does not imply weakness or selfishness. Instead, it shows self-respect and acceptance of one's limits. We do ourselves and others a favor by saying no because it enables us to be completely present and involved in the activities and relationships that are essential to us.

It is critical to establish limits and say no courteously and strongly. This entails communicating clearly and directly while still considering the needs and sentiments of others. For instance, we may say, "I appreciate your invitation, but I need to take some time for myself right now." We may maintain healthy connections with others while still prioritizing our well-being if we communicate our demands clearly and respectfully.

In conclusion, creating boundaries and saying no when required is critical to sustaining our general health and well-being. We may take charge of our lives and prioritize our happiness and satisfaction by defining our own needs and priorities and articulating them clearly and aggressively.

27. STAYING ORGANIZED AND KEEPING A TIDY LIVING SPACE

Keeping a clean and orderly living area may not be the first thing that comes to mind when we think of healthy habits, but it may greatly influence our emotional and physical well-being. A chaotic and congested environment may create tension, worry, and even physical injury. In this part, we will look at the advantages of remaining organized and practical techniques for decluttering and keeping a neat living area.

The Advantages of Staying Organized

Staying organized has been demonstrated in studies to offer several mental health advantages. Living in a crowded and chaotic environment may be stressful, causing worry and tension. A neat and orderly setting, on the other hand, may relax the mind and help us feel more in charge. Furthermore, organizing may boost productivity and keep us focused on our goals.

A clean living place may also be beneficial to one's physical well-being. Cluttered and unorganized environments may be dangerous, increasing the chance of accidents such as falls. We can move about more easily and lower the danger of accidents when we have a clean and orderly area.

Practical Tips for Organizing and Decluttering

Decluttering and organizing might seem to be a difficult process, but it does not have to be. We can create a useful and visually beautiful room by dividing the process into manageable parts.

Begin small: Decluttering a whole living area might be overwhelming. Instead, begin by addressing one area at a time. For example, start with a single closet or drawer and work up to bigger spaces.

Sort stuff into categories: Sort objects into categories such as retain, give, or throw as you declutter. This might help you remain organized and decide what to retain and what to discard.

Make a system: After you've decluttered, make a method for arranging your possessions. This includes the use of storage containers, shelves, and closet organizers. Having a specific spot for each thing will help you remain organized in the long term.

Maintain your area regularly: Maintaining your newly arranged environment regularly is important to prevent clutter from accumulating again. Set aside a few minutes each day to clean up and return objects to their proper locations.

Seek help: Decluttering and organizing may be difficult, particularly if you have considerable junk. Don't be hesitant to seek help from others. Consider asking friends or family members for assistance or hiring a professional organizer to get you started.

Keeping an orderly and clean living area may not seem an important element of a healthy lifestyle. Still, it may greatly influence our emotional and physical well-being. We may create a relaxing, useful, and safe environment by taking tiny actions to simplify and arrange our living environments. Incorporating this practice into our daily routine may help us feel more in control, boost our productivity, and improve our general well-being.

28. INSTEAD OF CAFFEINE OR SUGARY DRINKS, DRINK HERBAL TEA

Many depend on coffee or sugary drinks to help them through the day, yet these beverages may harm our health. Caffeine may produce jitters, anxiety, and sleep disruption, while sugary beverages can lead to weight gain and raise the risk of chronic illnesses like diabetes and heart disease. Herbal tea, on the other hand, offers a refreshing and healthful option that may help us feel better.

Herbal tea is caffeine-free and brewed using dried herbs, flowers, fruits, and spices. Chamomile, peppermint, ginger, and hibiscus are among popular herbal tea variations, each with a distinct taste and possible health advantages.

Chamomile tea, for example, is well-known for its relaxing effects and may aid in treating insomnia and anxiety. Peppermint tea is often used to treat digestive problems and headaches, and ginger tea may aid with nausea and inflammation. Hibiscus tea has a high concentration of antioxidants and has been demonstrated to decrease blood pressure.

Herbal tea may also help you remain hydrated by providing a tasty alternative to plain water. Staying hydrated is critical for sustaining good biological processes such as temperature regulation, joint lubrication, and digestive assistance. We may get dehydrated if we do not drink enough water. Symptoms include weariness, headaches, and dry skin.

Another advantage of drinking herbal tea is that it may be a healthy substitute for sugary beverages. Many individuals use sugary beverages regularly, such as soda, energy drinks, or fruit juices, which may result in weight gain and an increased risk of chronic illnesses. Herbal tea, on the other hand, is naturally low in calories and sugar, making it an excellent choice for people trying to reduce sugar consumption.

When selecting herbal tea, choosing high-quality products and carefully reading the labels is important. Some products may include artificial tastes or sweeteners, which might offset the possible health advantages. Furthermore, certain herbs might mix with drugs or have possible adverse effects, so it's advisable to consult with a healthcare expert if you have any concerns.

In conclusion, herbal tea is a tasty and healthful alternative to coffee or sugary beverages. It has several possible health advantages, including inducing relaxation and lowering the risk of chronic illnesses. To gain these advantages, choosing high-quality products, carefully reading labels, and consulting with a healthcare expert if necessary are important.

29. SELECTING WHOLE FOODS OVER PROCESSED FOODS

One of the most essential decisions you can make regarding eating a healthy diet is to favor natural foods over processed foods. Whole foods have been lightly processed or refined and are as near to their natural condition as possible. They are often richer in nutrients and fiber than processed foods and lower in added sugars, salt, and harmful fats. You may enhance your general health and lower your risk of chronic illnesses like heart disease, diabetes, and cancer by eating whole foods.

Whole foods include fruits and vegetables, whole grains, legumes, nuts and seeds, and lean proteins. These foods are all nutrient-dense, which means they have a high nutrient-to-calorie ratio. They are also fiber-rich, essential for maintaining digestion and avoiding chronic illness.

Processed foods, on the other hand, are often heavy in added sugars, salt, and harmful fats, which may lead to weight gain and other health concerns. They are also often deficient in minerals and fiber. Packaged snacks, candies, sugary beverages, white bread, spaghetti, and fast foods are all processed.

It is critical to prioritize diversity and balance while selecting whole foods. Consuming a mix of fruits, vegetables, whole grains, and proteins may assist to ensure you are obtaining a broad spectrum of nutrients. It's also critical to balance your macronutrient consumption (carbohydrates, protein, and fat) and prevent overeating.

Including whole foods in your diet may be simpler than you think. Here are some pointers to get you started:

Shop the perimeter of the Grocery store: Fresh vegetables, meat, and dairy products, all of which are whole foods, may be found here.

Examine food labels: Look for foods with few ingredients and avoid those with extra sugars, salt, and bad fats.

Cook at home: Cooking at home enables you to manage the ingredients and ensure that you utilize whole foods.

Replace processed snacks with whole food snacks: Snack on fruits, vegetables, nuts, or seeds instead of chips or cookies.

Experiment with new recipes: Experimenting with new recipes that use whole foods will help keep your diet interesting and gratifying.

Choosing natural foods over processed foods may improve your health and well-being significantly. By adopting one easy diet modification, you may enhance your nutrition, lower your risk of chronic illnesses, and feel better overall.

30. EATING FRUITS AND VEGETABLES WITH EVERY FOOD

One of the most essential healthy habits you can develop is to eat fruits and vegetables with every food. Fruits and vegetables are high in vitamins, minerals, fiber, and other nutrients necessary for good health. Unfortunately, many individuals do not regularly consume enough fruits and vegetables, which may result in vitamin shortages and other health issues. In this part, we'll look at the advantages of eating fruits and vegetables at every food and some recommendations for getting more of these items into your diet.

The Advantages of Eating Fruits and Vegetables at Every Food

Eating fruits and vegetables with every food offers several health advantages. Here are a few examples:

Improved Digestive Health: Fruits and vegetables are abundant in fiber, which aids in the smooth operation of your digestive system. Fiber also promotes fullness, which may help reduce overeating and encourage weight reduction.

Reduced Risk of Chronic Illnesses: Eating a fruit and vegetable-rich diet has been associated with a lower risk of chronic illnesses such as heart disease, diabetes, and obesity with certain cancers. These foods are high in antioxidants and other nutrients that help protect your cells from harm.

Better Mental Health: A diet high in fruits and vegetables has been linked to better mental health. This is most likely because these foods provide minerals crucial for brain function, such as folate and vitamin B6.

How to Include More Fruits and Vegetables in Your Diet

Adding extra fruits and vegetables to your diet might be difficult if you are not accustomed to eating them with every food. Here are some pointers to get you started:

Start Small: If you're not accustomed to eating fruits and veggies with every food, start with just one serving. You might, for example, include a banana in your breakfast, a salad in your lunch, and roasted veggies in your supper.

Experiment with Different Fruits and veggies: Eating the same fruits and veggies daily might get monotonous. To keep things interesting, try various types. Try new fruits and veggies or cook them differently than you have previously.

Keep Fruits and Vegetables on Hand: Keep fruits and vegetables on hand at all times to quickly include them in your foods. Keep a bowl of fruit and veggies on your kitchen counter to be ready to go when needed.

Sneak Them In: If you don't like fruits and veggies, try incorporating them into other foods. You could, for example, add spinach to a smoothie or puree veggies and mix them into spaghetti sauce.

Make Fruits and Vegetables the Stars: Fruits and vegetables don't have to be a side dish. Make them the center of attention by cooking foods with them as the primary element. You may, for example, cook a vegetable stir-fry or a fruit salad with yogurt and almonds.

Summary:

One of the most essential healthy habits you can develop is to eat fruits and vegetables with every food. These foods are high in vitamins, minerals, fiber, and other nutrients necessary for good health. You may enhance your digestive health, lower your risk of chronic illnesses, and improve your mental health by including more fruits and vegetables. Begin small, experimenting with various fruits and vegetables, keeping them on hand, sneaking them into other recipes, and making them the star of the show. With these recommendations, you can add more fruits and veggies to your diet and gain the advantages of this healthy habit.

31. INSTEAD OF BUTTER OR VEGETABLE OIL, USE OLIVE OIL OR COCONUT OIL

Cooking oil is a must-have in most kitchens, with several varieties to select from. Some oils are excellent for high-heat cooking, while others are ideal for salad dressings and marinades. Furthermore, certain oils are healthier than others, and switching to a better oil might result in considerable health advantages.

Olive oil and coconut oil are two common healthy cooking oil options. Both oils have been demonstrated to offer health advantages when used in moderation, and they are both useful in the kitchen.

Olive oil is produced by pressing olives, a common ingredient in Mediterranean cuisine. It contains monounsaturated fats, which have been demonstrated to decrease cholesterol and the risk of heart disease. Olive oil is also high in antioxidants, which aid in the prevention of inflammation and oxidative damage.

Extra virgin olive oil is ideal when cooking with olive oil since it is the least processed and maintains the greatest health advantages. Because extra virgin olive oil has a low smoke point, it should not be used in high-heat cooking. It's great for salad dressings, marinades, and low-heat cooking, including sautéing vegetables or creating soups and stews.

Coconut oil is produced by pressing the flesh of coconuts and has grown in popularity in recent years due to its health advantages. Coconut oil is high in medium-chain triglycerides (MCTs), a saturated fat that the body can readily absorb for energy. MCTs have been demonstrated to enhance metabolism, improve cognitive function, and decrease inflammation.

It is advisable to use unrefined, virgin coconut oil when cooking using coconut oil. It has a higher smoke point than extra virgin olive oil, making it ideal for high-heat cooking like frying or baking. Coconut oil may also be used instead of butter in baking recipes, adding a slight coconut flavor and making baked products moister.

It should be noted that although olive oil and coconut oil are both healthy alternatives, they should be used in moderation. Because both oils are rich in calories, they must be used carefully to prevent ingesting too many calories. Furthermore, they should be used with a healthy balanced diet rich in fruits, vegetables, whole grains, and lean meats.

In conclusion, substituting olive or coconut oil for butter or vegetables may provide considerable health advantages. Olive oil contains monounsaturated fats and antioxidants, while coconut oil has MCTs. When cooking with these oils, using them sparingly and in conjunction with a balanced diet is crucial. By switching to a healthier oil, you may enhance your general health and lower your risk of chronic illnesses.

32. TO SUPPORT GUT HEALTH, EAT PROBIOTICS-RICH FOODS LIKE YOGURT OR SAUERKRAUT.

Probiotics are live bacteria that improve human health, notably digestive and immunological function. They may be found in foods such as yogurt, kefir, sauerkraut, kimchi, and kombucha, as well as supplements. Probiotics have been demonstrated to be beneficial in treating various illnesses, including diarrhea, irritable bowel syndrome (IBS), and inflammatory bowel disease (IBD).

The gut microbiome is a microbial population that lives in the digestive system. These microbes are essential for digestion, food absorption, and immunological function. Dysbiosis, or imbalances in the gut microbiome, has been related to several health concerns, including autoimmune illnesses, obesity, and mental health difficulties.

By introducing helpful bacteria into the digestive tract, probiotics may assist in sustaining a healthy gut microbiota. They operate by colonizing the gut, pushing out dangerous bacteria, boosting the immune system, and increasing the function of the intestinal barrier.

Yogurt, which includes live cultures of Lactobacillus bulgaricus and Streptococcus thermophilus, is one of the most well-known sources of probiotics. Lactose, the sugar contained in milk, is broken down by these bacteria, making yogurt an excellent alternative for individuals who are lactose intolerant.

Sauerkraut, which is created by fermenting cabbage with lactic acid bacteria, is another probiotic-rich dish. These bacteria create lactic acid, which contributes to the sour taste of sauerkraut while also aiding in the preservation of the cabbage. Sauerkraut may be served as a side dish, mixed into sandwiches or salads, or even used as a pizza topping.

Kombucha is a fermented tea that contains probiotics. Sweet tea is fermented with a symbiotic culture of bacteria and yeast (SCOBY). Fermentation results in a tangy, somewhat sweet drink with various health advantages, including enhanced digestion and immunological function.

In addition to these foods, other probiotic supplements are on the market. These supplements are available in various formats, including capsules, powders, and liquids. Choosing a high-quality supplement with a range of helpful bacteria types is critical.

While probiotics may help with digestive and immunological health, it is crucial to remember that they are not a panacea. It is also important to keep a balance diet that includes a variety of fiber-rich fruits and vegetables, whole grains, and lean meats.

In conclusion, integrating probiotic-rich foods into your diet, such as yogurt, sauerkraut, and kombucha, may be an effective method to maintain gut health and increase immune function. Probiotics function by bringing good bacteria into the digestive tract, where they drown out harmful bacteria while supporting a healthy gut microbiota. Probiotic pills might also benefit those who do not get enough probiotics via their diet. However, before beginning any new supplement regimen, it is critical to maintain a balanced diet and consult with a healthcare expert.

33. EATING LESS MEAT AND EATING MORE PLANT-BASED PROTEIN SOURCES LIKE LEGUMES AND NUTS

Plant-based diets have grown in popularity in recent years due to their health advantages. One of the key reasons for this is a decrease in meat and animal products consumption, which has been related to several health issues such as heart disease, diabetes, and some forms of cancer. As a result, integrating more plant-based protein sources into your diet, such as legumes and nuts, may be an effective strategy to boost general health and well-being.

Legumes, which include beans, peas, and lentils, are high in plant-based protein, fiber, and other essential elements. Research has shown that eating beans regularly helps cut cholesterol, lessen the risk of heart disease, and improve blood sugar management. Furthermore, legumes are an inexpensive and sustainable food source, making them a perfect supplement to any diet.

Nuts are another excellent source of plant-based protein and healthy fats, fiber, and other essential elements. Consuming nuts regularly has been linked to a decreased risk of heart disease and enhanced cognitive function. Furthermore, since nuts can be readily included in foods and snacks, they are a handy and enjoyable option to enhance protein consumption.

While increasing plant-based protein sources might benefit general health, remember that not all foods are equal. Processed and high-fat plant-based foods, such as chips and sweets, should be eaten in moderation since they may lead to weight gain and other health issues.

When following a plant-based diet, it is also critical to obtain appropriate levels of all vital elements. To prevent shortages, plant-based sources of iron, calcium, and vitamin B12, for example, may need to be supplemented.

Eating less meat and more plant-based protein sources like legumes and nuts may be a simple and effective method to improve general health and well-being. You may gain the numerous advantages of a plant-based diet by including these items and paying attention to total nutrient intake.

34. EATING SMALL, FREQUENT MEALS THROUGHOUT THE DAY

Eating small, frequent meals throughout the day has become a popular weight reduction and metabolism-boosting method. This technique is based on the premise that eating smaller, more frequent meals may minimize hunger and cravings while keeping your metabolism at a consistent pace. However, the evidence for this method is conflicting, and it may not be the ideal option for everyone.

One of the primary advantages of eating small, frequent meals is that you may prevent overeating. You may control your appetite by eating every few hours and resisting consuming unhealthy snacks or huge foods. This is particularly beneficial for persons who suffer from cravings or emotional eating.

Eating small, regular meals may also help manage blood sugar levels. Long durations of fasting may cause blood sugar levels to plummet, resulting in weariness, irritation, and even migraines. You may prevent these symptoms by eating smaller meals daily and keeping your blood sugar levels constant.

However, other data shows that eating small, frequent meals may have negative consequences. Research published in the journal Nutrients, for example, discovered that although this technique may aid with weight reduction in the short term, it may not be sustainable in the long run.

Long-term Participants in the research who ate small, frequent meals for six months gained weight, probably due to increased nibbling and grazing throughout the day.

Furthermore, eating small, frequent meals may leave some individuals dissatisfied or continuously hungry. This might be because smaller foods are less full than bigger ones or deficient in specific nutrients. Pay attention to your body's hunger cues and change your food plan as necessary.

Overall, eating small, frequent meals may benefit certain individuals, particularly those who suffer from overeating or blood sugar management. It may not be the ideal method for everyone, so listen to your body and choose a food plan that works for you.

Summary: Eating small, frequent meals throughout the day might benefit weight reduction and metabolic improvement. It may aid in the regulation of blood sugar levels and the prevention of overeating. However, the evidence for this method is varied, and it may not be long-term sustainable. It is important to listen to your body and develop a diet plan that works for you.

35. TO KEEP MEALS INTERESTING, TRY NEW RECIPES AND CUISINES.

A healthy, well-balanced diet is critical for general health and well-being. Many individuals, however, struggle to maintain good eating habits because of boredom or a lack of variety in their foods. Trying different dishes and cuisines to make foods fresh and exciting is one method to fight this.

One advantage of experimenting with various dishes and cuisines is learning about diverse cultures and customs via food. This might broaden your culinary horizons and expose you to new tastes and ingredients. Trying new recipes may also be a creative and exciting outlet, enabling you to experiment with various ingredient combinations and culinary methods.

Trying different recipes and cuisines might have health advantages besides the fun component. You may ensure a wide assortment of nutrients by combining fruits, vegetables, healthy grains, and lean meats into your foods. This may benefit general health and help avoid vitamin shortages.

Consider studying and seeking inspiration from other cultures and places to introduce new foods and cuisines into your diet. Look for recipes online or in cookbooks; don't be afraid to experiment.

To go outside of your comfort zone. You may also experiment with mixing new ingredients into existing foods to give them a new spin.

Keep portion proportions and overall food balance in mind when experimenting with new recipes. While experimenting with new tastes and ingredients is fun, it's still vital to have a balanced diet with the right amount of protein, carbs, and healthy fats.

Experimenting with various dishes and cuisines may be a fun and tasty approach to maintaining a healthy, balanced diet. You may broaden your culinary horizons and add diversity to your foods by studying various cultures and customs via food. Remember to keep portion proportions and general balance in mind, and don't be afraid to experiment in the kitchen.

36. SAVORING EACH BITE AND EATING MINDFULLY

Eating mindfully and appreciating each food is a healthy practice that may have various physical and mental health advantages. Mindful eating entails paying attention to the food we consume, our bodily feelings, and our emotional condition when we eat. It entails being fully present in the moment, free of distractions and judgments, and creating a feeling of curiosity and openness.

In studies, mindful eating has been found to aid with weight control, digestion, and general health. We are more conscious of our hunger and fullness signals when we eat mindfully, which may help us avoid overeating and promote better digestion. We also eat healthier and have a higher appreciation for the flavor and texture of our foods.

Furthermore, mindful eating has been related to mental health benefits such as decreased stress, anxiety, and sadness. Being more present and aware when eating allows us to connect more intimately with our bodies and emotions, cultivating self-compassion and acceptance.

To begin practicing mindful eating, create a quiet setting for foods. These are all examples of this: turning off devices, setting the table, and taking a few deep breaths before dining. It's also crucial to take your time and appreciate each mouthful, paying attention to the food's tastes, textures, and scents.

Paying attention to our bodily feelings while eating may also help us tune in to our hunger and fullness signals. This is frequently checking in with our body throughout the food and quitting when we are content rather than when the plate is empty or too full.

Being conscious of our emotional condition while eating is another part of mindful eating. This includes recognizing any stress, worry, or unhappiness that may influence our eating behaviors and devising appropriate coping strategies. For example, taking a few deep breaths or practicing gratitude before eating might help us feel more focused and relaxed.

In conclusion, mindful eating and enjoying each mouthful may be effective for changing our relationship with food and enhancing our general health and well-being. We may tune in to our bodily and emotional signals, make better eating choices, and create a feeling of self-compassion and acceptance by being present and aware as we eat.

37. AVOIDING ARTIFICIAL SWEETENERS AND HIGH-FRUCTOSE CORN SYRUP

Artificial sweeteners like high-fructose corn syrup (HFCS) are widely found in processed foods and drinks. While they are often touted as better alternatives to sugar, there is mounting evidence that they may be harmful to human health.

Aspartame and sucralose, two artificial sweeteners, are often used as sugar alternatives in diet and low-calorie goods. However, research suggests they may interfere with our bodies' normal hunger and satiety signals, leading to overeating and weight gain. Furthermore, the use of various artificial sweeteners has been associated with an elevated risk of type 2 diabetes, metabolic syndrome, and cardiovascular disease.

HFCS is a highly refined sugar often found in soda, juice, other sweetened drinks, and processed foods such as candy and baked goods. Consumption of high fructose corn syrup has been related to an increased risk of obesity, type 2 diabetes, and other health problems. One explanation is that HFCS may not be as effective as natural sugars in signaling fullness, causing people to take more calories than they need.

To limit your consumption of artificial sweeteners and HFCS, read food labels carefully and eat as many whole, unprocessed foods as possible.

Look for goods naturally sweetened with fruit or honey, minimal quantities of natural sugar, or a natural low-calorie sweetener such as stevia.

Water is always the greatest option when it comes to beverages. If you prefer sweetened beverages, try preparing your own at home using natural ingredients such as fruit or herbs. If you must drink soda or other sugary beverages, try to restrict your consumption and provide smaller servings.

In conclusion, eliminating artificial sweeteners and high-fructose corn syrup may be a significant step toward a healthy diet. You may decrease your consumption of these potentially dangerous components and improve your general health and well-being by eating whole, unprocessed foods and carefully reading labels.

38. REDUCING ADDED SUGARS IN YOUR DIET

One of the most essential actions you can take toward improved health is reducing your added sugar intake. While sugar is a natural and important component of our foods in the form of glucose, which our cells utilize for energy, added sugars — those added to foods and beverages during processing — have been associated with several poor health effects.

Many processed foods have added sugars, including baked products, candies, soft drinks, and sweet beverages. They may aggravate obesity, type 2 diabetes, and other chronic disorders. Furthermore, excessive sugar consumption may result in tooth damage, vitamin shortages, and a compromised immune system.

Begin by reading food labels and ingredient lists to decrease your consumption of added sugars. Search for phrases such as "sugar," "syrup," "cane juice," "dextrose," and "fructose." All of these are signs of added sugars. Even "healthy" items, such as many granola bars and flavored yogurts, may include additional sugars.

Focus on complete, unprocessed foods instead. Without the additional sugars, fruits, veggies, nutritious grains, and lean meats may all fulfill your sweet taste. Instead of sugary drinks, consume water or unsweetened liquids such as tea or coffee.

Look for methods to lessen the quantity of sugar asked for in a recipe, whether cooking or baking. Try replacing part of the sugar in baked products with applesauce or mashed bananas. You may also try natural sweeteners like honey or maple syrup in moderation.

Remember that finding a balance that works for you is more important than eliminating sugar. Small modifications made over time may lead to significant benefits for your health.

To summarize, reducing added sugars is a vital step toward improved health. You may reduce sugar consumption and enhance your general well-being by reading food labels, concentrating on whole foods, and limiting sugar in your cooking and baking.

39. INSTEAD OF PROCESSED SNACKS, EAT HEALTHY SNACKS LIKE NUTS, FRUIT, OR VEGETABLES.

Eating nutritious snacks may be an essential part of maintaining a healthy diet. Snacking may assist in satisfying hunger, minimize overeating at foods, and offer essential nutrients throughout the day. Not all snacks, however, are made equal. Processed snacks, such as chips, cookies, and candies, are often heavy in calories, sugar, and harmful fats, with little nutritious benefit. On the other hand, snacking on nuts, fruit, or vegetables may deliver critical nutrients such as fiber, protein, and vitamins.

The influence on overall health is one of the most significant advantages of selecting nutritious snacks. A diet rich in fruits and vegetables has been demonstrated in studies to lower the risk of chronic illnesses such as heart disease, stroke, and some forms of cancer. Furthermore, snacking on nuts may deliver crucial healthy fats that can help minimize the risk of heart disease.

Another advantage of healthy snacking is the effect it has on weight control. Eating nutritious snacks might help you avoid overeating at foods, reducing total calorie consumption. Furthermore, snacking on high-protein nuts or fiber-rich fruits and vegetables might help boost feelings of fullness and satiety, decreasing snacking overall.

When selecting healthy snacks, it is important to consider nutritional content and portion size. While fruits and vegetables are typically healthy choices, keeping portion sizes in mind is crucial to prevent overeating. A big apple, for example, may have up to 100 calories, so keep this in mind when planning snacks throughout the day. Similarly, although nuts may be a healthy snack option, they are also heavy in calories, so moderation is essential.

Planning ahead of time is one approach to making healthy eating simpler. Having nutritious snacks on hand might help you avoid reaching for processed snack alternatives when hungry. Here are some examples of healthy snack options:

- Apples, bananas, and berries are examples of fresh fruit.
- Raw veggies like carrots, celery, and cucumbers.
- Almonds, walnuts, and pumpkin seeds are examples of nuts and seeds.
- Yogurt made using Greek yogurt or cottage cheese
- Hummus or guacamole with whole-grain crackers

Regarding healthy snacking, keeping nutritional content and portion sizes in mind is crucial. Incorporating nutritious snacks into a well-balanced diet may benefit general health and weight control.

40. FOOD PREP FOR TIME-SAVING AND HEALTHY EATING HABITS

Food preparation has recently grown popular to save time while maintaining healthy eating habits. The concept is simple: prepare foods beforehand to have fresh, nutritious food on hand when needed. You can resist the urge to eat fast food or order takeout, which is heavy in calories, harmful fats, and salt. Instead, you may have a wonderful and well-balanced dinner to benefit your health and well-being.

One of the primary advantages of food preparation is that it might save you time. You may remove the need to cook daily by devoting a few hours each week to food preparation. This is particularly useful for those who don't have the time or energy to cook after a hard day at work. All you have to do with pre-prepared dishes is reheat and serve.

Another advantage of food planning is that it might assist you in maintaining good eating habits. You are less likely to seek unhealthy snacks or fast food when you have nutritious foods readily accessible. Food planning also allows you to regulate portion proportions and avoid food waste. By planning your foods ahead, you can guarantee that you only purchase what you need and use up items before they go bad.

Having a strategy in place is critical before you begin food planning. Begin by deciding the dishes you want to create and the required servings. You may then create a grocery list and shop for the essential goods. Regarding food planning, picking ingredients that will last a long time is important. Soups and stews, for example, are simple to freeze, as are items that can be kept in the fridge for many days, such as roasted vegetables or grilled chicken.

Set aside time to make your foods after you have all the components. This might include slicing veggies, preparing meats, or putting together foods in containers. You may then refrigerate or freeze your foods until you're ready to consume them.

It's critical to keep food safety in mind during food planning. To avoid contamination, wash your hands and utensils before handling food and store your foods in sealed containers. Following appropriate storage standards is also critical to keep your food fresh and safe to consume.

To summarize, food preparation is an excellent approach to save time while maintaining good eating habits. You may guarantee that you always have nutritious food accessible when you need it by planning and preparing foods ahead of time. Food planning may be a great tool in your healthy living toolkit, whether you're a busy professional or just want to eat more healthfully.

41. INSTEAD OF SUGARY DRINKS OR SODA, DRINK HERBAL TEA OR WARM WATER WITH LEMON.

One of the simplest methods to boost your health is to substitute herbal tea or warm water with lemon for sugary beverages or soda. Sugary beverages are well-known causes of weight gain, obesity, and type 2 diabetes. Drinking herbal tea or warm water with lemon not only helps to minimize sugar consumption but it also has several health advantages.

Herbal teas are produced from leaves, flowers, roots, and bark. They include antioxidants, vitamins, and minerals that may assist in promoting general health and are caffeine-free. Chamomile tea, for example, has been demonstrated to have relaxing effects that help decrease stress and encourage relaxation. In contrast, green tea has been shown to offer several health advantages, such as boosting brain function, lowering the risk of heart disease, and even supporting weight reduction.

Warm water with lemon is also an excellent substitute for sugary beverages. Lemon has a high concentration of vitamin C and antioxidants, which may stimulate the immune system and promote skin health. Additionally, lemon water may assist with digestion and cleansing and balance the body's pH levels.

One of the primary advantages of drinking herbal tea or warm water with lemon is that it may help minimize sugar consumption. Sugary beverages are rich in calories and have been linked to weight gain and obesity. Consuming sugary beverages frequently, according to research published in the American Journal of Clinical Nutrition, may contribute to weight gain and an increased risk of type 2 diabetes. Individuals may dramatically lower their sugar consumption and enhance their general health by substituting sugary beverages with herbal tea or warm water with lemon.

In addition to lowering sugar consumption, sipping herbal tea or warm water with lemon will help you stay hydrated. Water is required for the body to operate correctly, and dehydration may cause various health issues such as headaches, exhaustion, and constipation. Drinking herbal tea or warm water with lemon will help you drink more water and stay hydrated, enhancing your general health and well-being.

Another advantage of drinking herbal tea or warm water with lemon is that it helps aid digestion. Herbal drinks like ginger and peppermint have been shown to have anti-inflammatory qualities that may help with digestive disorders, including bloating, gas, and nausea. Lemon water may also assist with digestion by stimulating the synthesis of digestive enzymes.

In conclusion, drinking herbal tea or warm water with lemon is a simple but effective strategy to promote general health.

Individuals may dramatically decrease their sugar intake by substituting these healthy options for sugary beverages. Herbal teas and lemon water also provide a variety of health advantages, such as improving digestion, lowering stress, strengthening the immune system, and supporting weight reduction. Including herbal tea or warm water with lemon in your daily routine may improve your health and well-being.

DRINKING ALCOHOL IN MODERATION OR NOT AT ALL

Alcohol use is common during social and cultural occasions. However, drinking in excess may be harmful to one's health. Excessive alcohol use has been linked to liver disease, heart disease, stroke, cancer, and mental health concerns, among other things, according to the Centers for Disease Control and Prevention (CDC). As a result, it is important to weigh the hazards and advantages of alcohol intake to evaluate if it is a healthy habit to develop.

According to the Dietary Guidelines for Americans, moderate alcohol intake is defined as up to one drink per day for women and up to two drinks per day for men. A normal drink includes 14 g of pure alcohol, which is similar to 12 oz. of beer, 5 oz. Of wine or 1.5 oz. of distilled spirits. Moderate alcohol use has been linked to a lower risk of cardiovascular disease, type 2 diabetes, and some malignancies, including breast and colon cancer. Furthermore, moderate alcohol intake has been demonstrated to raise HDL, or "good" cholesterol, which may aid in the prevention of heart disease.

The advantages of moderate alcohol usage, however, must be balanced against the hazards. Even average alcohol intake may raise the risk of certain health problems, such as high blood pressure, liver disease, and cancers of the mouth, throat, liver, and breast. Furthermore, alcohol use might impair drug effectiveness, increase the likelihood of accidents and injuries, as well as contribute to addiction and alcoholism. Pregnant women and anyone with specific medical problems, such as liver illness or a history of addiction, should abstain from alcohol entirely.

It is important to remember that alcohol use affects people differently based on characteristics such as age, weight, gender, and heredity. As a result, it is critical to check with a healthcare expert to decide if drinking alcohol is safe and healthy for one's specific circumstances. Furthermore, it is essential to consume alcohol wisely and in moderation, avoiding exceeding the permitted limits or drinking while driving.

In conclusion, moderate alcohol intake may provide health advantages, such as lowering the risk of heart disease and type 2 diabetes. Still, these benefits must be balanced against the hazards of alcohol consumption, such as liver disease, cancer, and addiction. Moderation and appropriate intake, like any dietary habit, are essential for sustaining good health. Individuals should, thus, contact a healthcare expert to establish if alcohol use is safe and acceptable for their specific situation.

43. CHOOSE WHOLE GRAINS OVER REFINED GRAINS

Choosing whole grains over processed grains is one of the simplest and most powerful nutritional improvements you can make. Whole grains include the full-grain kernel, including the bran, germ, and endosperm, while refined grains remove the bran and germ, leaving just the starchy endosperm. Many of the minerals and fiber contained in whole grains are removed during this process, making refined grains a less healthy alternative.

Studies have demonstrated that whole grains have several health advantages. Research published in the American Journal of Clinical Nutrition, for example, found that persons who consumed three servings of whole grains per day had a 20% reduced risk of heart disease than those who consumed less than one serving per week. Another research published in the Journal of Nutrition found that eating whole grains decreased the risk of developing type 2 diabetes.

Consuming whole grains may aid weight control and lower the risk of chronic illnesses. This is due to the fiber in whole grains, which may help you feel full and satisfied, lowering your chances of overeating. According to research published in the Journal of Nutrition, those who ate whole grains had a lower BMI and were less likely to be overweight or obese than those who ate refined grains.

So, how do you make the transition to whole grains? When shopping for bread, pasta, rice, and other grain-based items, search for whole-grain choices. To simplify identifying goods, many now carry a "whole grain" label. However, it is important to carefully read the label since some goods may include a combination of whole and refined grains.

Consider substituting whole grains for refined grains in your favorite dishes when cooking at home. For example, use whole-grain pasta instead of white pasta in your spaghetti food, and in your stir-fry, use quinoa or brown rice instead of white rice.

If you're not used to them, it may take some time to become acclimated to the taste and texture of whole grains. Begin by including tiny quantities of whole grains in your foods, gradually increasing the quantity over time. This might help you adjust to the flavor and texture while enjoying your favorite foods.

Eating whole grains rather than processed grains is a simple yet effective dietary shift that may give several health advantages. By making this transition, you may minimize your risk of chronic illnesses, help in weight control, and enhance your general health and well-being.

44. EATING LEAN PROTEIN SOURCES LIKE CHICKEN OR FISH

A healthy diet should include lean protein sources such as chicken or fish. Protein is necessary for the body's tissue growth and repair and helps us feel full and satisfied after foods. However, not all protein sources are created equal, and choosing lean choices to promote overall health is critical.

Chicken breast is an excellent source of lean protein. Chicken breast is low in fat and calories while rich in protein, making it an excellent option for people trying to gain or maintain muscle mass. It's extremely adaptable since it may be prepared in several ways, including grilling, baking, and sautéing.

Fish is yet another great source of lean protein. Fish strong in omega-3 fatty acids, such as salmon, tuna, and mackerel, are helpful to heart health and cognitive function. Fish is also rich in protein and low in saturated fat, making it an excellent option for general health.

When selecting protein sources, consider not just their protein level but also their entire nutritional worth. Processed meats, such as deli meat and sausage, are rich in salt and preservatives and may raise the risk of certain health problems. Red meat, although rich in protein, is also heavy in fat. When ingested in excess, it is heavy in saturated fat and may raise the risk of heart disease.

Protein vegetarian or vegan foods, such as beans, lentils, and tofu, are also wonderful choices. These foods are rich in protein and fiber while lower in calories and fat than animal-based protein sources. They also include a range of other minerals, such as iron and zinc, which benefit general health.

It is extremely simple to include lean protein sources in your diet. Begin by including chicken breast or fish in your foods a few times weekly. To keep things interesting, use new cooking techniques and flavors. For vegetarians and vegans, consider including plant-based protein sources such as beans, lentils, and tofu in foods.

In addition to selecting lean protein sources, portion sizes must be considered. While protein is essential to a balanced diet, too much of a good thing may be harmful. Protein consumption recommendations vary by age, gender, and activity level but usually range from 0.8-1.2 grams of protein per kilogram of body weight. It's also crucial to consider the overall balance of your diet and to incorporate a range of nutrient-dense foods, including fruits, vegetables, whole grains, and healthy fats.

In conclusion, including lean protein sources in your diet is vital to a healthy lifestyle. Chicken breast and fish are wonderful alternatives, as are vegetarian and vegan protein sources such as beans and tofu. When selecting protein sources, consider not just their protein level but also their entire nutritional worth. And, like with everything else in life, moderation is essential. Pay attention to portion sizes and aim for a well-balanced diet rich in nutrient-dense foods.

45. EATING BREAKFAST EVERY DAY TO GET YOUR METABOLISM STARTED

One of the most essential healthy habits you can form is eating breakfast daily. A good breakfast jumpstarts your metabolism, gives you energy for the day, and may even help you maintain a healthy weight. In this part, we will explain why breakfast is so essential, what a nutritious breakfast looks like, and how to include breakfast into your daily routine.

First, let us discuss why breakfast is so vital. Your body has been fasting for many hours when you get up in the morning. Breakfast aids in breaking the fast and jumpstarting your metabolism for the day. According to research, breakfast eaters are more likely to maintain a healthy weight and have better overall health than breakfast skippers. Eating breakfast may also help you feel more awake and focused throughout the day by improving cognitive function and mood.

Let's have a look at what a nutritious breakfast looks like. A balanced food should contain a variety of carbs, protein, and healthy fats. Carbohydrates offer energy, protein aids in the formation and repair of tissues, and healthy fats keep you full and happy. All nutritious breakfast dishes include whole grain bread with avocado and a poached egg, porridge with nuts and berries, or a smoothie prepared with Greek yogurt, fruit, and spinach.

It's critical to understand that not all breakfast items are made equal. Sugary cereals and pastries, for example, might be heavy in calories but poor in nutrients. These foods may contribute to weight gain and other health concerns by causing a drop in energy levels later in the day. When selecting breakfast items, look for healthy foods that are minimally processed and high in nutrients.

So, how can you include breakfast in your daily schedule? If you're not accustomed to having breakfast, starting small and gradually working your way up to a full food might be beneficial. Start with a piece of fruit or a tiny dish of yogurt in the morning and gradually increase the amount of food as you get used to eating breakfast. You may also make overnight oats or a breakfast casserole to heat up in the morning.

If you're pressed for time in the morning, there are many quick and simple breakfast alternatives. Some examples are a peanut butter and banana sandwich, a smoothie prepared with frozen fruit and Greek yogurt, or a breakfast burrito with scrambled eggs, vegetables, and salsa.

In conclusion, having breakfast daily is a critical healthy habit that may kickstart your metabolism, offer energy, and enhance your general health. A balanced food should contain a variety of carbs, protein, and healthy fats. When selecting breakfast items, look for healthy foods that are minimally processed and high in nutrients. If you aren't used to having breakfast, Begin with a modest portion and gradually increase to a full food. Even if you're pressed for time in the morning, there are plenty of quick and simple breakfast alternatives.

46. PACKING A HEALTHY LUNCH INSTEAD OF EATING OUT

Bringing your lunch from home is one of the most easy and efficient strategies to improve your nutrition while saving money. Eating out often consumes more calories, salt, and harmful fats than if you brought your own lunch. Furthermore, bringing your lunch gives you greater control over the quality and amount of your foods, making it simpler to keep to your health goals. Here are some healthy lunch-packing ideas:

Plan: Spend some time planning your lunches at the start of each week. This will save you time and money while ensuring that you have healthy alternatives.

Use leftovers: Cook extra and utilize the leftovers for lunch the following day if you're preparing supper. This is an excellent approach to decrease food wastage while still ensuring a nutritious, prepared food.

Focus on whole foods: Pack your lunch with nutritious foods such as fruits, veggies, whole grains, and lean protein. These foods will provide important nutrients while keeping you full and content throughout the day.

Avoid processed foods: Skip the packaged snacks and processed foods, which are often heavy in salt, sugar and unhealthy fats. Instead, choose whole foods that will fuel your body.

Invest in a good lunch container: Ensure you have a high-quality container to keep your food fresh and warm. Look for leak-proof, microwave-safe, and easy-to-clean containers.

Pack snacks: Pack nutritious snacks such as cut-up vegetables, fruit, almonds, or yogurt to keep you satiated throughout the day. This will also assist you in avoiding unhealthy vending machine choices.

Don't forget about hydration: Remember to bring a reusable water bottle to remain hydrated during the day. Avoid sugary beverages in favor of water or herbal tea.

By bringing a nutritious lunch, you may keep on track with your health goals while saving money. It's simple to prepare nutritious foods that nourish your body and keep you feeling fantastic with a little thought and preparation.

47. AVOIDING FAST FOOD AND CONVENIENCE MEALS

Because of their convenience and accessibility, fast food and convenience meals have grown in popularity. However, these foods are often rich in calories, harmful fats, and salt, and they frequently lack critical elements required for a balanced diet. In this part, we'll talk about why it's important to avoid fast food and convenience meals and some strategies for selecting better eating choices.

The Dangers of Fast Food and Convenience Meals

Fast food and convenience meals are often heavy in calories, bad fats, and salt, which may result in weight gain and various health issues. These foods are often highly processed and include added sugars, artificial flavors, and preservatives, which may harm one's health. Fast food intake has been related to an increased risk of obesity, type 2 diabetes, heart disease, and other chronic disorders in studies.

Fast food and convenience meals may be addicting in addition to being harmful. They are often rich in sugar and salt, which may contribute to cravings and overeating. This may lead to a vicious cycle of bad eating behaviors that is difficult to quit.

Making Healthier Food Selections

Planning and preparing foods at home is one of the greatest ways to avoid fast and convenient meals. This might be difficult for individuals with demanding schedules, but it is a crucial step toward better overall health. When cooking at home, using complete, nutrient-dense foods high in vitamins and minerals is important.

Here are some pointers to help you make healthy dietary choices:

Make a plan: Make weekly time to plan your foods and snacks. When you're hungry and in a hurry, this may help you resist the temptation of fast food and convenience meals.

Choose whole foods: Choose whole foods that are minimally processed and high in nutrients, such as fruits, vegetables, whole grains, lean protein sources, and healthy fats.

Cook at home: Cooking at home gives you control over the components in your foods, ensuring that they are wholesome and nutritious.

Pack your food: Make nutritious snacks to take with you on the road. This might assist you in resisting the lure of unhealthy snacks and fast foods.

Read labels: When shopping for packaged goods, read the labels for added sugars, other unhealthy fats and salt. Select items with little additional ingredients.

Keep portion sizes in mind: Even nutritious foods may be hazardous if taken in excess. Pay attention to portion sizes and your body's hunger and fullness cues.

By implementing these easy dietary modifications, you may minimize your consumption of harmful fast food and convenience foods while improving your general health and well-being.

Summary:
While fast food and convenience foods are handy, they are often unhealthy, leading to weight gain and various health concerns. You may make better food choices and minimize your consumption of fast food and convenience foods by planning, selecting whole foods, cooking at home, bringing snacks, reading labels, and being conscious of portion sizes. This may result in better overall health and well-being.

48.   SLOW EATING AND THOROUGH CHEWING OF FOOD

Eating slowly and carefully is a simple but effective practice that may significantly improve your digestive health and general well-being. We are more prone to develop digestive disorders such as bloating, gas, and indigestion when we eat hastily or do not chew our food correctly. Furthermore, we may also not absorb nutrients, resulting in inadequacies and other health issues.

According to research, eating slowly and thoroughly may enhance digestion and nutritional absorption. By chewing your food, you enable your saliva to combine with it and start digestion. This may aid in the breakdown of carbs and other nutrients, making them simpler for your body to absorb.

Eating slowly may also help you tune in to your body's natural hunger and fullness cues. Because it takes time for your brain to detect that you are full, eating too rapidly may cause you to overeat before your brain has a chance to catch up. Eating slowly and thoroughly may help you realize when you're full, reduce overeating, and promote good weight control.

According to one research, individuals who ate slowly consumed fewer calories and felt fuller after foods than those who ate rapidly. Slow eaters also exhibited lower levels of specific appetite-regulating hormones, indicating that eating slowly may help manage hunger and satiety.

Slow and thoughtful eating may help produce a more comfortable and pleasurable food experience. We may not completely enjoy the tastes and textures of our food when we eat fast or on the run. We might feel more fulfilled and nourished if we take the time to taste and appreciate each food.

It is easy to include this practice into your everyday routine. Put your fork or spoon down between bites, take deep breaths, and concentrate on the tastes and sensations of your food. Avoid distractions like TV or your phone and concentrate on the current moment and the dining experience.

In conclusion, eating slowly and thoroughly may offer a variety of advantages for your digestive health, weight control, and general well-being. You may support good digestion, minimize overeating, and enhance your connection with food by taking the time to appreciate your food and listen to your body's natural cues. Take a deep breath, calm down, and relish each mouthful the next time you dine.

49. TRYING INTERMITTENT FASTING OR TIME-RESTRICTED EATING

Intermittent fasting (IF) and time-restricted eating (TRE) are two prominent ways to manage when and how much we eat. Both have received attention in recent years as prospective weight loss, metabolic health, and inflammation-reduction treatments.

Intermittent fasting entails alternating between eating and fasting intervals. The 16/8 approach, the 5:2 diet, and alternate-day fasting are all methods to practice IF. The 16/8 approach, which entails eating inside an 8-hour window and fasting for the other 16 hours, is the most common.

In contrast, time-restricted eating restricts the amount of time you spend eating daily. For example, you may eat all your foods within a 10-hour window and then fast for the next 14 hours.

Both IF and TRE may aid calorie reduction, contributing to weight loss. They may also increase insulin sensitivity, lower blood pressure, and decrease inflammation.

One study published in the journal Cell Metabolism found that a 12-hour TRE schedule (i.e., eating within a 12-hour window and fasting for the remaining 12 hours) improved insulin sensitivity and reduced liver fat in overweight men with prediabetes. Another study published in the New

England Journal of Medicine found that alternate-day fasting (i.e., fasting every other day) improved markers of cardiovascular health in healthy adults.

While these findings are encouraging, it is crucial to highlight that IF and TRE may not be suitable for everyone, before considering IF or TRE, pregnant or nursing women, persons with a history of disordered eating, and those with specific medical issues should visit a healthcare professional.

Furthermore, many people may not find IF and TRE feasible or pleasurable. Some individuals may struggle to keep to a rigorous eating schedule, while others may suffer severe side effects such as weariness, headaches, or irritability when fasting.

Overall, IF and TRE are two techniques for limiting when and how much we eat that can benefit our health. However, before adopting these strategies, like any dietary or lifestyle change, speak with a healthcare physician and listen to your body to decide what works best for you.

50. AVOID EATING LATE AT NIGHT OR CLOSE TO BEDTIME

Many individuals have difficulty with late-night nibbling or eating close to sleeping. Consuming foods late at night, whether due to boredom, stress, or habit, may harm physical and mental health. In this part, we will look at why avoiding eating late at night is crucial and provide suggestions for breaking the habit.

One of the most important reasons to avoid eating late at night is that it might interfere with sleep. Consuming foods close to bedtime might cause gastric acid production to rise, causing heartburn and interfering with the body's normal sleep cycle. Furthermore, eating late at night may produce blood sugar spikes, contributing to agitation and restlessness.

Another reason not to nibble late at night is that it might lead to overeating and weight gain. When people are weary and unable to make good decisions, they eat more calories at night. Furthermore, the body's metabolism slows at night. Thus, calories taken late at night are more likely to be stored as fat.

It might be difficult to break the habit of eating late at night, but numerous ways can help. First, it is critical to understand the factors contributing to late-night eating. Stress, boredom, and weariness are all common causes. Once you've determined, you can focus on establishing healthy coping skills if you know your triggers. For example, if stress is a trigger, consider doing deep breathing exercises or taking a warm bath before bed instead of grabbing food.

Another way to minimize late-night munching is to arrange your foods and snacks in advance. When you have healthy alternatives, you're less likely to seek junk food or convenience foods late at night. Pack a nutritious snack before bedtime, such as a piece of fruit or a handful of almonds.

Having a calm nighttime ritual that does not include eating is also beneficial. This might be taking a hot bath, reading a book, or engaging in meditation or yoga. By developing a routine, you may instruct your body to connect nighttime with relaxation rather than food.

Finally, while you strive to eliminate the habit of eating late at night, be patient and forgiving with yourself. It takes time and work to change behaviors, and setbacks are common. Don't berate yourself if you indulge in a late-night snack. Instead, use it as a chance to learn and improve your plan.

Eating late at night or close to sleep benefits physical and mental health. Late-night munching may cause sleep disruption, overeating, and weight gain. Determining the causes of late-night eating is essential to quit the habit. Prepare for stressors, set a calming nighttime ritual, and be gentle with yourself. You may create healthy habits that benefit your well-being by making little adjustments over time.

51. EATING A VARIETY OF COLORS AND TEXTURES IN YOUR MEALS

Eating a variety of colors and textures in your meals is an important part of maintaining a balanced diet. You may ensure that you are obtaining the nutrients your body needs by incorporating a variety of fruits, vegetables, whole grains, and lean meats.

When it comes to fruits and vegetables, it is important to choose a variety of hues. Because various produce colors suggest different sorts of nutrients, having a rainbow of colors in your foods will help you acquire a variety of vitamins, minerals, and antioxidants. Dark leafy greens, such as spinach and kale, are high in calcium and vitamin K, while orange vegetables, such as carrots and sweet potatoes, are high in beta-carotene and vitamin C.

Textures, in addition to colors, should be considered. Including different textures in your foods might help you feel more content while providing several health advantages. Fiber-rich foods like whole grains and legumes may help you feel fuller for longer and promote digestive health.

Experiment with various fruits and vegetables to include various colors and sensations in your foods. Try incorporating a new veggie into your stir-fry or roasting a colorful array of vegetables as a side dish. Include whole grains in your diet in a variety of forms. Try several methods to cook grains, including quinoa, brown rice, and whole wheat pasta.

Consider plant-based protein sources such as beans, lentils, tofu, and lean meats such as chicken and fish. Changing up your protein sources may help you acquire a variety of nutrients as well as environmental and ethical advantages.

You may guarantee that you obtain the nutrients your body needs by concentrating on diversity in your diet. Adding various colors and textures to your foods may also make healthy eating more fun and rewarding.

Eating a variety of colors and textures in your foods is an essential part of maintaining a balanced diet. Because various fruits and vegetables have different sorts of nutrients, having a variety of colors in your foods may help you acquire a variety of vitamins, minerals, and antioxidants. Textures, in addition to colors, should be considered. Experimenting with various fruits, veggies, whole grains, and proteins will assist you in discovering new and interesting ways to eat healthily. You may guarantee that you obtain the nutrients your body needs by concentrating on diversity in your diet.

52. EATING ANTIOXIDANT-RICH FOODS TO PROTECT AGAINST OXIDATIVE STRESS

Eating antioxidant-rich foods is a vital component of a healthy diet. Antioxidants are substances that aid in protecting our cells against oxidative stress, which is generated by damaging molecules known as free radicals. Free radicals are naturally formed in our bodies due to metabolism, but they may also be produced by environmental pollutants such as air pollution and cigarette smoke. When free radicals build up in our bodies, they may cause cell damage and contribute to the development of chronic illnesses such as cancer, heart disease, and Alzheimer's.

Fortunately, several foods strong in antioxidants may help protect our cells from oxidative stress. Fruits, vegetables, nuts, seeds, and whole grains are excellent sources of antioxidants. These foods are high in antioxidants such as vitamins A, C, and E and other substances such as carotenoids and flavonoids.

Eating various colorful fruits and vegetables is one of the greatest methods to increase your antioxidant intake. Antioxidants are especially abundant in brightly colored fruits such as berries, leafy greens, and bell peppers. Berries like blueberries, strawberries, and raspberries are particularly high in anthocyanins, a kind of antioxidant that has been demonstrated to have potent anti-inflammatory and anti-cancer qualities.

Nuts and seeds are also rich sources of antioxidants. Nuts such as almonds, walnuts, and pecans are high in vitamin E, but seeds such as chia and flax are high in lignans, which have been linked to a lower risk of breast cancer. Whole grains like oats and quinoa are also high in antioxidants and other essential elements like fiber and minerals.

In addition to consuming antioxidant-rich foods, you should limit your exposure to free radicals. This includes avoiding cigarette smoke and other environmental contaminants and limiting your intake of processed and fried foods, which may emit hazardous substances when cooked at high temperatures.

In conclusion, eating antioxidant-rich foods is a vital aspect of a balanced diet. These substances may aid in the protection of our cells from oxidative stress, which can lead to the development of chronic illnesses. Consuming a range of colorful fruits and vegetables, nuts, seeds, and whole grains is an excellent approach to guaranteeing enough antioxidant intake. To reduce your intake of damaging free radicals, you should limit your exposure to environmental contaminants and processed foods.

53. AVOIDING TRANS FATS FOUND IN FRIED AND BAKED GOODS

Trans fats, or trans fatty acids, are unsaturated fats in various processed foods, including fried dishes, baked products, and snacks. These fats have been related to a variety of health issues, including cardiovascular disease, diabetes, and obesity. Consequently, avoiding trans fats is a crucial healthy habit in your daily routine.

Trans fats are formed when liquid oils are hydrogenated, which converts them to solid fats. These boosts processed goods' shelf life and taste stability, making them popular in the food sector. Consuming trans fats, on the other hand, may have a variety of detrimental health repercussions. Trans fats may raise LDL (bad) cholesterol levels while lowering HDL (good) cholesterol levels, increasing the risk of heart disease. They've also been connected to a higher risk of type 2 diabetes and obesity.

To avoid trans fats, it is critical to read food labels carefully. The FDA mandates that the quantity of trans fats be included on the Nutrition Facts label of all packaged goods. Look for foods that have no trans fat per serving. Be aware, however, that a food may be labeled "trans-fat-free" if it contains fewer than 0.5 grams of trans fat per serving. Check the ingredients list for hydrogenated or partly hydrogenated oils to ensure you are not ingesting trans fats.

Choose healthy cooking oils such as olive, avocado, or coconut oil while cooking at home. Solid fats, such as shortening or margarine, are generally high in trans fats. Choose natural, healthy foods like fruits, vegetables, and lean meats. These foods are not only trans-fat-free, but they also include critical nutrients that promote general wellness.

To summarize, avoiding trans fats is a critical healthy practice that may help lower the risk of heart disease, diabetes, and obesity. Read food labels attentively and eat natural, whole foods as much as possible. You may enhance your health and well-being over time by making tiny modifications to your diet.

54. INSTEAD OF SALT, USE SPICES AND HERBS TO FLAVOR FOOD

We are increasingly turning to healthier food options as we become more conscious of the influence of our foods on our overall health. One of the most important aspects of a healthy diet is lowering salt consumption. Excess sodium may lead to high blood pressure and other health issues, so finding alternatives to salt to taste our food is critical. One of the greatest ways to enhance flavor without adding salt is by using herbs and spices.

Herbs and spices have been used in cooking for generations for both taste and medical purposes. Herbs and spices, in addition to contributing taste, may give various health advantages. Ginger, for example, has anti-inflammatory effects, while garlic may aid in cholesterol reduction.

There are several ways to use herbs and spices in your cuisine. Other common options include Basil, rosemary, thyme, oregano, cumin, coriander, and cinnamon. You may add depth and complexity to your recipes by combining various herbs and spices to produce a broad spectrum of tastes, from spicy to sweet.

Using herbs and spices to flavor your cuisine may be cheaper than purchasing pricey pre-packaged seasonings. Created seasoning combinations that typically include excessive quantities of salt. You can be certain that you obtain the highest quality components for your dishes if you use fresh herbs and spices.

To begin incorporating herbs and spices into your cuisine, try experimenting with various taste combinations to see what works best. For example, consider combining thyme, rosemary, and garlic for a traditional taste profile in a chicken food. Add chili flakes, paprika, or cayenne pepper to your foods to heat them.

Another fantastic method to use herbs and spices in your cooking is to create marinades, dressings, and sauces. Making your dressings and sauces allows you to manage the quantity of salt and other ingredients in your foods, ensuring they are as nutritious as possible.

To summarize, flavoring your food with herbs and spices is a healthy and enjoyable way to lower salt consumption. Herbs and spices add depth and complexity to your dishes and may also give various health advantages. You may change your foods into a delightful and nutritious eating experience by experimenting with various flavor combinations and introducing herbs and spices.

55. TO SUPPORT BONE HEALTH, EAT CALCIUM-RICH FOODS LIKE DAIRY OR LEAFY GREENS.

Calcium is important in maintaining bone health and strength, an important element of general health and well-being. As a result, enough quantities of calcium-rich foods must be consumed as part of a balanced diet.

Calcium is a mineral required for several body activities, such as muscular contraction, neuron function, and blood coagulation. However, the most well-known function of calcium is its involvement in bone health. Calcium is a fundamental component of bone tissue that contributes to bone strength and shape.

When there is a calcium deficit, the body will draw calcium from the bones, weakening bones and an increased risk of fractures. This is why eating calcium-rich foods is essential for bone health.

Calcium is abundant in dairy products such as milk, cheese, and yogurt. One cup of milk has around 300 milligrams of calcium, but one serving of yogurt contains approximately 150 milligrams of calcium. Cheese is a rich source of calcium as well.

1 ounce of cheddar cheese contains about 200 milligrams of calcium. However, not everyone can eat dairy products due to

lactose sensitivity or other factors. Fortunately, people who cannot drink dairy may get calcium in other ways. Calcium is abundant in leafy green foods such as spinach, kale, and collard greens. One cup of cooked spinach has around 250 milligrams of calcium, while one cup of cooked kale contains approximately 100 milligrams of calcium.

Tofu, walnuts, and fortified plant-based milk are other calcium-rich non-dairy options. A half-cup of tofu has around 250 milligrams of calcium, while a quarter-cup of almonds contains approximately 95 milligrams of calcium. Plant-based milk, such as soy or almond milk, may provide up to 300 milligrams of calcium per cup.

Other variables, such as vitamin D consumption, exercise, and some drugs, also impact calcium absorption. Because vitamin D aids in calcium absorption, eating vitamin D-rich foods or taking supplements as needed is important. Regular activity, especially weight-bearing activities such as walking, jogging, or weight lifting, also aids in bone density and strength maintenance.

In conclusion, eating calcium-rich foods is essential for bone health. Calcium is abundant in dairy products, but non-dairy sources such as green leafy vegetables, tofu, walnuts, and fortified plant-based milk are other good choices. When attempting to maintain healthy bones, it is important to consider other variables that impact calcium absorption, such as vitamin D consumption and exercise. Individuals may promote their bone health and general well-being by including calcium-rich foods in a balanced diet and participating in regular exercise.

56. TO SUPPORT HEART HEALTH, EAT FOODS HIGH IN OMEGA-3 FATTY ACIDS.

Eating foods rich in omega-3 fatty acids has been linked to various health advantages, notably cardiovascular health. Omega-3 fatty acids are a form of polyunsaturated fat required by the body for various tasks. It cannot, however, create them on its own; thus, they must be received from nutrition.

Omega-3 fatty acids are classified into three types: alpha-linolenic acid (ALA), eicosapentaenoic acid (EPA), and docosahexaenoic acid (DHA). Plant-based sources of ALA include flaxseeds, chia seeds, and walnuts. EPA and DHA are found mostly in fatty fish like salmon, tuna, and mackerel.

Consuming foods rich in EPA and DHA has been demonstrated in studies to have a substantial influence on heart health. Individuals who eat a diet rich in omega-3 fatty acids have a decreased risk of heart disease and stroke than those who consume a diet low in omega-3s, according to studies. Omega-3 fatty acids have been found to aid in reducing inflammation in the body, a recognized risk factor for heart disease.

Omega-3 fatty acids have also improved various risk factors for heart disease. They have been found, for example, to help decrease triglyceride levels in the blood, which is another risk factor for heart disease. Furthermore, omega-3 fatty acids may lower blood pressure, which is another risk factor for heart disease.

While eating fatty fish is the most well-known source of omega-3s, it is not the only method to get these critical fatty acids. Plant-based ALA sources may potentially be good for heart health. However, it is crucial to remember that the conversion rate of ALA to EPA and DHA in the body is rather low. As a result, consuming a mix of plant-based ALA sources and fatty fish sources of EPA and DHA may be advantageous. Individuals should take at least two fatty fish foods weekly to receive enough EPA and DHA. Omega-3 supplements may be a realistic choice for those not eating seafood. However, supplement usage should be discussed with a healthcare professional since supplements may interact with certain drugs and are not appropriate for everyone.

In conclusion, eating foods with omega-3 fatty acids may have considerable heart health advantages. Omega-3 fatty acids have been found to decrease inflammation, cut triglyceride levels, and may aid in blood pressure control. While fatty fish is the most well-known source of omega-3 fatty acids, plant-based ALA sources may also be helpful. To maintain optimal consumption of omega-3s, eating a variety of plant-based and fatty fish sources is critical. Individuals who do not eat fish might consider omega-3 supplements but should consult a healthcare physician first.

57. TO SUPPORT ENERGY LEVELS, EAT IRON-RICH FOODS LIKE RED MEAT OR SPINACH.

Iron is a necessary mineral that is important to the human body. It is involved in forming red blood cells, which transport oxygen throughout the body. The body cannot manufacture enough red blood cells without adequate iron, resulting in iron deficiency anemia. This may lead to weariness, weakness, and other health issues.

Dietary iron is classified into two types: heme iron and non-heme iron. Heme iron is present in animal-based foods such as red meat, poultry, and fish and is easier for the body to absorb than non-heme iron. Plant-based iron sources include beans, lentils, spinach, and fortified cereals.

While both forms of iron are necessary, people adopting a vegetarian or vegan diet must be extra careful to get adequate iron-rich foods. This is because non-heme iron is more difficult for the body to absorb, and vegetarians and vegans may not ingest as much iron as meat eaters.

Increased energy levels are one of the primary advantages of eating iron-rich foods. Iron is required to create hemoglobin, the protein in red blood cells that transports oxygen to the body's tissues. The body cannot function without adequate iron. Inadequate hemoglobin production causes weariness and weakness.

Among the top sources of iron-rich foods are:

Red meat: Heme iron is abundant in beef, hog, lamb, and other forms of red meat.

Poultry: Chicken and turkey are also high in heme iron.

Fish and seafood: Oysters, clams, and other shellfish contain a lot of iron.

Beans and lentils: These plant-based foods are abundant in fiber, other vital minerals, and non-heme iron.

Spinach and other leafy greens: These vegetables are high in non-heme iron and vitamins and minerals such as vitamin C, which may aid in iron absorption.

Fortified grains: Many cereals, breads, and other grains are fortified with iron to help individuals obtain more of this crucial vitamin.

It is also vital to know that eating too much iron might be dangerous. While the body needs iron, excessive quantities may cause constipation, nausea, and liver damage. Consuming iron-rich foods as part of a balanced and diverse diet is essential, as is speaking with a healthcare practitioner if you have concerns about your iron consumption.

In conclusion, eating iron-rich foods is vital for maintaining energy levels and general health. Iron is found in red meat, chicken, fish, beans, lentils, spinach, and fortified cereals. While it is essential to take adequate iron, it is equally critical to avoid taking too much iron. Individuals may improve their health and well-being by incorporating iron-rich foods in a diverse and balanced diet.

58. EATING VITAMIN C-RICH FOODS TO SUPPORT IMMUNE FUNCTION

"An apple a day keeps the doctor away," the adage goes. It turns out that there is some truth to that phrase, particularly when it comes to strengthening your immune system. Vitamin C is one of the most critical elements for immune function; luckily, it can be found in various delectable foods.

Vitamin C is a water-soluble vitamin that helps the body's immune system by promoting the creation and function of white blood cells, which aid in the fight against infections and disorders. Furthermore, vitamin C is a potent antioxidant that aids in the protection of cells from damage caused by dangerous chemicals known as free radicals.

Citrus fruits such as oranges, lemons, and grapefruits, as well as kiwifruit, strawberries, and papaya, are excellent sources of vitamin C. Broccoli, cauliflower, Brussels sprouts, and bell peppers are other good suppliers of this essential component.

It is simple and tasty to include these items in your diet. Start your day with a glass of freshly squeezed orange juice or a smoothie prepared with kiwifruit and strawberries. Slice up some bell peppers and serve them with hummus for a nutritious snack. Hummus or guacamole are two options. For supper, roast a pan of mixed veggies, such as broccoli, cauliflower, and Brussels sprouts, and serve with your preferred protein source.

It is crucial to emphasize that vitamin C is necessary for immune function but is not a panacea for preventing sickness. Maintaining a healthy diet and lifestyle, getting adequate sleep, and maintaining excellent hygiene are all critical components of immune system maintenance.

In addition to eating vitamin C-rich foods, you may want to consider taking a vitamin C supplement. However, it's always a good idea to consult your doctor before beginning any new supplement routine since certain supplements may interfere with prescriptions or have negative effects.

Vitamin C is a vital nutrient for immune function and disease prevention. You may assist in boosting your body's natural defenses and remain healthy by including vitamin C-rich foods in your diet.

59. DRINKING GREEN TEA FOR IT'S ANTIOXIDANT AND HEALTH BENEFITS

Green tea has been consumed for millennia and is one of the world's most popular drinks. It is derived from the Camellia sinensis plant's leaves. It is high in antioxidants, which help protect the body from damage caused by dangerous molecules called free radicals. In this part, we'll go over the health advantages of green tea, its possible role in illness prevention, and how to include it in your daily routine.

Green tea's strong antioxidant content is one of its key advantages. In particular, it is high in catechins, a kind of antioxidant that has been demonstrated to help lower the risk of chronic illnesses such as cancer and heart disease. Green tea also includes caffeine, which may assist in boosting brain function and alertness.

Green tea may also assist in enhancing heart health, according to research. Green tea, in particular, has been shown in studies to help lower levels of "bad" LDL cholesterol, which may contribute to the development of heart disease. Green tea has also been demonstrated to enhance blood vessel function, which may help lower the risk of cardiovascular disease and stroke.

Green tea offers potential weight reduction and control advantages. Specifically, green tea includes catechins, which may aid in boosting metabolism and fat burning. Green tea has also been demonstrated to help suppress appetite, which may help individuals eat fewer calories and lose weight.

Regarding illness prevention, studies have shown that green tea may help lower the risk of some forms of cancer. Green tea drinkers, in particular, may have a decreased chance of acquiring breast, prostate, and colorectal cancers, according to research. More study, however, is required to properly grasp the potential advantages of green tea in cancer prevention.

Green tea may be simple and tasty to include in your everyday routine. Brewing a cup of hot tea using loose tea leaves or tea bags is a simple method to enjoy green tea. To make an iced tea, boil it and chill it before adding ice. Green tea may also be used in many dishes, including smoothies, as a foundation for marinades and salad dressings.

While green tea is usually considered harmless for most people, it does contain caffeine, which may induce anxiety, irritation, and sleeplessness in some people. Furthermore, green tea may interfere with some drugs, so if you are on any prescription medications, you should consult your healthcare provider before introducing green tea into your regimen.

In conclusion, green tea is a pleasant and healthful beverage that may provide several health advantages. There are several reasons to consider including green tea in your daily routine, ranging from its high antioxidant content to its possible function in illness prevention and weight control. Just consult with your doctor before making any big dietary or lifestyle changes.

60. GETTING ENOUGH VITAMIN D FROM THE SUN OR SUPPLEMENTS

Vitamin D has received much attention in health and well-being in recent years. It is an essential ingredient that aids calcium absorption, promotes bone health, and has been linked to various other health advantages. Vitamin D is a unique substance that our bodies may produce in reaction to sunshine exposure. However, many individuals do not acquire enough vitamin D from sunlight alone due to various variables such as lifestyle choices, skin color, and geographical location. In this part, we'll look at the necessity of obtaining enough vitamin D, the dangers of vitamin D insufficiency, and how you acquire enough vitamin D via sunlight or pills.

The recommended daily vitamin D consumption varies according to age, gender, and health condition. Adults should consume 600-800 IU of vitamin D each day, according to the National Institutes of Health (NIH). Some studies, however, show that many individuals may need greater doses to reach adequate vitamin D levels. A blood test that measures 25-hydroxyvitamin D [25(OH)D] in your blood is the best technique to establish your vitamin D status.

A lack of vitamin D has been related to various health issues, including bone abnormalities, autoimmune illnesses, infections, and certain malignancies. Severe vitamin D deficiency in children may result in Rickets, a disease that causes brittle bones, slowed development, and skeletal malformations. Vitamin D insufficiency in adults may lead to osteomalacia, a disorder characterized by weak bones, muscular weakness, and an increased risk of fractures.

The sun is our bodies' principal source of vitamin D. When our skin is exposed to sunshine, it creates vitamin D3, which is subsequently processed in the liver and kidneys into the active form of vitamin D. However, various variables such as the time of day, season, latitude, and cloud cover may all have an impact on our bodies' capacity to generate vitamin D. Furthermore, many individuals spend the majority of their time inside, wear clothing that covers the majority of their skin, or use sunscreen to protect their skin from UV damage, all of which may lower vitamin D production.

Supplements may be a useful strategy to guarantee appropriate vitamin D levels, especially for people who get little sun or are at risk of shortage. There are two vitamin D supplements: vitamin D2 (ergocalciferol) and vitamin D3 (cholecalciferol). Vitamin D3 is favored since it is easier for the body to absorb and use. Supplements are available in various dosages, and it is important to choose the optimum amount depending on your specific requirements and health state. Choosing a recognized brand and following the manufacturer's use guidelines is also critical.

In conclusion, enough vitamin D intake is critical for general health and well-being. Vitamin D shortage may cause various health concerns; thus, it is critical to get enough vitamin D levels by sunlight, supplements, or a mix of both. A blood test is the best method to establish your vitamin D level, and it is critical to contact your healthcare professional before beginning any vitamin D supplementation. You may take a proactive step toward preserving good health and wellness by deliberately acquiring adequate vitamin D.

61. EATING FIBER-RICH FOODS TO SUPPORT DIGESTIVE HEALTH AND REGULARITY

Fiber is an important ingredient frequently disregarded in our diets, yet it is needed for digestive health and regularity. Fiber is a carbohydrate that the body cannot digest. Therefore, it goes through the digestive system mostly undigested. This is why fiber is so beneficial to our health.

Fiber is classified into two types: soluble and insoluble. In the digestive system, soluble fiber dissolves in water, creating a gel-like material. This form of fiber aids in the digestion of foods and may aid in regulating blood sugar levels. Insoluble fiber, on the other hand, does not dissolve in water and hence adds weight to the stool, promoting regularity.

Whole grains, fruits, vegetables, beans, and nuts are all fiber-rich. These foods are rich in fiber and high in other nutrients that are beneficial to general health. Including additional fiber in your diet may provide many health advantages. Fiber, for example, may help lower the risk of constipation, hemorrhoids, and diverticulitis. It may also help decrease cholesterol, minimize the risk of heart disease, and manage blood sugar levels, which is crucial for people with diabetes.

It is critical to gradually increase your fiber intake while drinking lots of water. This may assist in avoiding discomforts like bloating and gas. It is also crucial to remember that certain people, such as those with inflammatory bowel disease, may need to restrict their consumption of particular forms of fiber.

Adding extra fiber to your diet is a simple yet effective strategy to improve digestive health and regularity while also increasing overall health and well-being. You may get the various advantages of fiber by eating a range of high-fiber foods and gradually increasing your consumption.

62. EAT PROBIOTICS-RICH FOODS OR TAKE SUPPLEMENTS TO SUPPORT GUT HEALTH

A healthy stomach is critical to overall health and fitness. The gut microbiota, which includes bacteria, viruses, and fungi, is home to billions of microorganisms. The microbiota in the gut is important for digestion, nutritional absorption, and immunological function. It also aids in the control of infections and the creation of important vitamins and neurotransmitters.

Consuming probiotic-rich foods or taking probiotic supplements is one strategy to improve gut health. Probiotics are living bacteria that give health advantages to the host when taken in sufficient quantities. These helpful bacteria aid in maintaining a healthy microbial balance in the gut, facilitating good digestion and immunological function.

Probiotics may be found in fermented foods such as yogurt, kefir, sauerkraut, kimchi, and tempeh. These foods are fermented naturally, which stimulates the development of healthy bacteria. When ingested regularly, these foods may help enhance gut health and lower the risk of certain illnesses.

Probiotic supplements are also readily accessible and may help promote gut health. Specific strains of helpful bacteria have been found to give health advantages in these supplements. To guarantee safety and effectiveness, however, choosing a high-quality supplement from a renowned manufacturer is essential.

In addition to probiotics, it is critical to consume prebiotic-rich foods to promote the development of beneficial bacteria in the gut. Prebiotics are fibers that are not digested in the small intestine and instead feed beneficial bacteria in the colon. Prebiotics are abundant in garlic, onions, leeks, asparagus, bananas, and whole grains.

Consuming probiotic-rich foods or taking probiotic supplements has been demonstrated in studies to provide several health advantages. Studies have shown probiotics to help lessen the symptoms of irritable bowel syndrome, boost immunological function, and even lower the risk of some forms of cancer.

However, it is crucial to realize that not all probiotics are made equal. Distinct types of bacteria have distinct health advantages, and the effects of probiotics might vary from person to person. It is critical to choose a probiotic supplement with a specific strain of bacteria that has been demonstrated to give health benefits for a certain ailment.

In conclusion, keeping a healthy stomach is critical to overall health and fitness. Probiotic-rich foods and supplements may assist in maintaining gut health by encouraging the development of beneficial bacteria. It is also critical to eat prebiotic-rich foods to promote the development of beneficial bacteria. It is critical to pick a high-quality probiotic supplement from a recognized manufacturer and a specific strain of bacteria that has been demonstrated to give health benefits for a certain ailment.

63. DRINKING WATER BEFORE, DURING, AND AFTER EXERCISE TO STAY HYDRATED

Staying hydrated is critical for overall health and well-being, particularly while participating in physical activity. When you exercise, your body loses water via sweating; if you don't replace that water, you risk dehydration, which may induce weariness, dizziness, and even heatstroke. That is why drinking water before, during, and after exercise is important.

Drinking water before exercise helps your body prepare for physical exertion. This is particularly critical if you are exercising in hot and humid weather. Drinking water before exercise helps to keep your body hydrated, which may help reduce cramps and other discomforts throughout your activity.

It is essential to drink water during exercise to replenish the fluids lost via sweat. You may need to drink more or less water depending on the intensity and length of your exercise. Drink around 17 to 20 ounces of water two to three hours before activity and then another 8 ounces every 20 to 30 minutes throughout your workout.

It's important to drink water after exercise to assist your body recover and rehydrate. You may feel dizzy if you do not restore the fluids you lost throughout your exercise. You'll feel tired and sluggish, and you may not be able to perform well in your next exercise. Drinking water after exercise helps your body recover faster by replacing lost fluids.

When exercising, it is essential to consider electrolytes in addition to water. Electrolytes are minerals that are lost via sweat and serve to maintain fluid balance. You may need to replace your electrolytes and water if you are doing high-intensity activity or working out in hot and humid weather. You may accomplish this by drinking sports drinks or eating electrolyte-rich foods like bananas, avocados, and coconut water.

In conclusion, being hydrated before, during, and after exercise is critical for good health and well-being. Water before exercise helps prepare your body for physical exertion, while water during exercise helps restore lost fluids. Drinking water after exercise aids in the recovery and rehydration of your body. When exercising, keep electrolytes in mind, particularly in hot and humid environments or during high-intensity activity. Staying hydrated can help you perform at your best throughout your exercises while keeping you healthy.

64. TO PREVENT INJURY, STRETCH BEFORE AND AFTER EXERCISE.

Stretching is an important part of physical exercise since it helps avoid injury and improves flexibility. Stretching as part of your training program may also improve athletic performance and mobility. In this part, we'll look at the advantages of stretching before and after exercise and give some pointers on stretching correctly.

There are two forms of stretching: static stretching and dynamic stretching. Static stretching is retaining a stretch for an extended length of time, and dynamic stretching is going through a range of motion to warm up the muscles before activity. Although both stretching methods may be useful, dynamic stretching is often suggested before exercise since it helps prepare the body for movement and minimizes the chance of injury.

Stretching before exercise may aid flexibility, range of motion, and injury prevention. Stretching before exercise warms up your muscles and prepares them for physical action. This may aid in the prevention of muscular strains and other ailments. Stretching also enhances sports performance by improving range of motion and flexibility. This may help you move more smoothly and efficiently during physical activities.

Stretching after exercise is also beneficial in preventing muscular pain and stiffness. Muscles become tight and constricted as you work out. Stretching after exercise can help relax your muscles and keep them from stiffening and getting painful. Stretching after exercise may also help you increase your flexibility and range of motion, which can help you avoid injury and enhance your athletic performance over time.

It is essential to stretch correctly to prevent damage. Warm up your muscles by doing modest aerobic exercises like running in place or jumping jacks. Then, slowly and gently stretch, holding each stretch for 15-30 seconds. To prevent muscular imbalances, stretch all sides of your body evenly. Avoid bouncing or jerking during stretches since this might result in harm.

In conclusion, stretching before and after exercise is vital to a healthy lifestyle. It may aid in the prevention of injury, the improvement of flexibility and range of motion, and the enhancement of athletic performance. Stretching as part of your fitness program may help you remain healthy and active for years.

65. DOING CARDIO AND STRENGTH TRAINING EXERCISES TO IMPROVE OVERALL FITNESS

Participating in cardio and strength training routines is essential to obtain total fitness. Cardiovascular exercise, usually known as cardio, is any activity that boosts heart rate and blood circulation. Such activities include running, cycling, swimming, and even brisk walking. On the other hand, strength training uses weights or resistance to grow muscle and improve strength.

Cardiovascular activities benefit cardiovascular health by strengthening the heart and increasing blood flow. Furthermore, cardio helps to burn calories and reduce body fat, which may result in a healthy body weight and a lower chance of chronic illnesses like diabetes, heart disease, and cancer.

Strength training activities, on the other hand, aid in the development of muscle mass and the enhancement of general strength. This may assist in improving posture, balance, and stability, as well as promoting bone density, which can aid in the prevention of osteoporosis. Strength exercise may also boost metabolism and enhance overall body composition by reducing fat and boosting muscular mass.

A mix of cardio and strength training routines may bring several health advantages. Examples include improved cardiovascular health, greater muscular growth and strength, enhanced bone density, and reduced body fat. Furthermore, by offering a range of various workouts, mixing these exercises may assist in reducing boredom and enhance overall motivation.

It is critical to begin a fitness regimen initially and gradually increase the intensity and length of the activities. This may aid with injury prevention and general fitness improvement over time. It is also important to choose workouts suitable for one's fitness level and to change the routines to avoid boredom and maintain general fitness.

In conclusion, combining cardio and strength training routines may bring several advantages for general fitness. These workouts may help enhance cardiovascular health, muscular mass and strength, bone density, and body fat. When beginning a fitness regimen, it is important to start cautiously and gradually raise the intensity and length of the workouts and choose exercises suited to one's fitness level.

66. TRYING NEW EXERCISES OR FITNESS CLASSES TO KEEP WORKOUTS INTERESTING

Regular physical exercise is essential for general health and well-being. However, many people find it difficult to stick to a continuous fitness plan owing to boredom or a lack of desire. To tackle this problem, try different activities or fitness programs to keep workouts fresh.

When it comes to fitness, variety is vital. Individuals may target various muscle groups, enhance cardiovascular health, and avoid burnout by participating in various activities. Trying new hobbies may also be a great way to challenge the body and push beyond physical limits.

When it comes to discovering new activities or fitness programs, there are several alternatives. Yoga, Pilates, kickboxing, and spin classes are all available at many gyms and fitness facilities. These sessions provide an organized setting with competent teachers, making it a good choice for people who are new to a certain sport.

Individuals may also engage in outdoor activities such as hiking, kayaking, and rock climbing. These sports not only give a physical challenge but also enable people to appreciate nature and unplug from the worries of daily life.

Several internet tools are accessible for people who want to work out at home. Many fitness instructors offer virtual lessons that may be seen from the comfort of your own home. Now, many fitness applications are available that provide planned exercises and assistance to people of all fitness levels.

Remembering that attempting new activities or fitness programs might be scary, particularly for individuals new to physical activity, is vital. However, remember that everyone needs to start somewhere and that growth takes time and persistence. Individuals should pay attention to their bodies and begin with pleasant and attainable activities. To guarantee perfect form and technique, it is also essential to seek help from competent teachers or trainers.

To summarize, experimenting with different exercises or fitness courses is a good method to keep workouts fresh, avoid fatigue, and push the body. Among the many possibilities, individuals may discover activities that suit their interests and fitness level. Individuals may enhance their general health and well-being by introducing diversity into their workout program.

67. GETTING OUTSIDE AND EXERCISING IN NATURE

Physical activity and exercise have long been recognized as beneficial to health and well-being. Regular exercise may help lower the risk of chronic illnesses, including heart disease, diabetes, and obesity. However, exercising outside in nature may bring advantages that indoor exercise cannot.

Being in nature has been demonstrated in studies to improve mental health by lowering stress and anxiety, enhancing mood and self-esteem, and improving cognitive performance. Furthermore, outdoor exercise has been linked to better satisfaction and desire to continue exercising compared to indoor exercise.

Hiking, jogging, cycling, swimming, and even gardening are all great ways to include outdoor fitness. The natural surroundings give a sensory experience that may enhance the enjoyment and engagement of exercise. Being outside may also create a connection to the environment and develop awareness and presence.

Furthermore, due to the natural terrain and weather conditions, outdoor exercise might be harder and more diverse than indoor exercise. Jogging on a path, for example, might give different amounts of slope and topography than jogging on a treadmill. Additionally, because of the uneven terrain and barriers, outdoor exercise may give a larger range of motion and train more muscle groups.

It is important to remember that while indulging in outdoor exercise, care must be taken to protect oneself from the weather and any threats. Wearing adequate clothes and footwear, utilizing sunscreen, keeping hydrated, and being aware of possible animal or terrain risks are all precautions.

Overall, including outdoor activity in your regimen may bring several health advantages besides indoor exercise. Individuals may enhance their physical and mental health while enjoying the beauty and peace of nature by taking advantage of their surroundings and adding physical exercise.

68. USING RESISTANCE BANDS OR BODYWEIGHT EXERCISES FOR AT-HOME WORKOUTS

Although the advantages of exercise are widely established, not everyone has the time or means to visit a gym. Fortunately, there are efficient methods for obtaining a fantastic work out in the privacy of your own home.

Resistance bands and bodyweight workouts are two popular methods for meeting fitness objectives without leaving the home. Resistance bands are low-cost, adaptable exercise equipment that may target every major muscle group. They are available in several resistance levels, allowing you to choose the band that best suits your fitness level. Resistance bands may be used for workouts, including bicep curls, tricep extensions, squats, and lunges. They're also excellent for stretches and mobility exercises.

Bodyweight workouts are another great approach to increasing strength and endurance without equipment. Because these workouts utilize your body weight as resistance, you may practice them anywhere and anytime. Push-ups, sit-ups, squats, lunges, and planks are bodyweight exercises. You may build a full-body workout that challenges your muscles and raises your heart rate by mixing various activities.

Resistance bands and bodyweight exercises have the benefit of being low-impact, which means they are less likely to cause joint discomfort or damage when compared to high-impact workouts like jogging or jumping. This makes them an excellent choice for seniors or joint pain patients.

Another benefit is that they are very adaptive. Resistance bands may be modified by varying their length or utilizing various bands with varying resistance levels. Bodyweight exercises may be altered by adjusting the angle, range of motion, or pace. You may keep challenging yourself and avoid plateauing in your fitness improvement.

It is critical to begin a resistance band or bodyweight training regimen cautiously and with appropriate technique. It is also important to warm up before exercise and cool down afterward. Several internet tools may help you practice workouts effectively and securely.

In conclusion, resistance bands and bodyweight exercises are excellent at-home training choices for increasing strength, endurance, and mobility. Because they are low-impact, adaptive, and versatile, they are appropriate for individuals of all fitness levels and ages. You may attain your fitness objectives without leaving the home if you include these workouts into your regimen.

69. EXERCISING WITH A FRIEND OR FAMILY MEMBER FOR ACCOUNTABILITY AND MOTIVATION

Regular exercise is a vital component of living a healthy lifestyle. Physical exercise lowers the risk of chronic illnesses and improves mental and general well-being. On the other hand, maintaining a steady fitness practice may be difficult, especially when one lacks desire. Exercising with a friend or family member may help you overcome these obstacles since it gives you the accountability and inspiration you need to maintain a fitness plan.

There are various advantages to having a workout companion. To begin with, working out with a friend or family member may be a lot of fun. It allows you to catch up, chat, and connect while participating in a healthy exercise. This may make exercise less of a task and a pleasant activity to look forward to. Having a workout partner may also make the process of exercising more fun by providing a feeling of camaraderie and support. This may be especially advantageous for people with difficulty exercising alone or staying motivated independently.

Exercising with a partner may also create a feeling of accountability. When we make promises to others, we are more likely to keep them. A workout buddy depending on us to show up and put in the effort may be a tremendous motivation to continue a regular fitness regimen. It also gives a healthy feeling of competitiveness as we seek to stay up with our partner's success and push ourselves to achieve new heights.

Exercising with a partner may help us improve our form and technique in addition to giving responsibility and incentive. It is beneficial to have someone spot us during weightlifting exercises or offer comments on our form during yoga or Pilates to ensure we complete activities properly and securely. This may aid in injury prevention and ensure we get the most out of our activities.

When working out with a partner, there are a few things to remember. First and foremost, we must locate someone who shares our fitness objectives and talents. When we have differing fitness levels, it may be difficult to find challenging and pleasant activities for us. Similarly, locating someone dependable and devoted to maintaining a regular fitness regimen is critical. Workout partners that are erratic or unpredictable may rapidly become a source of irritation and impair our development.

In conclusion, exercising with a friend or family member may be an excellent strategy to overcome the problems of sticking to an exercise regimen. It gives responsibility, incentive, and a feeling of community, which may make exercise less of a task and more of a pleasurable experience. When looking for an exercise partner, look for someone with fitness objectives and talents comparable to yours and who is dedicated to keeping to a regular workout regimen. We may attain our fitness objectives and get the numerous advantages of a healthy lifestyle with the appropriate partner.

70.   LISTENING TO MUSIC OR AN AUDIOBOOK DURING WORKOUTS TO MAKE THEM MORE ENJOYABLE

Physical exercise may greatly influence our general health and well-being if we include it in our daily routine. On the other hand, working out may be a monotonous and repetitious chore that many people detest. Fortunately, there are methods to make physical exercise more pleasurable, one of which is listening to music or audiobooks while exercising.

According to research, listening to music while exercising may improve performance by enhancing mood and decreasing perceived effort. One research discovered that listening to music while working out may boost endurance by up to 15%. This is because music may distract us from the pain we may experience during exercise, enabling us to push ourselves harder and for longer lengths of time.

Audiobooks, on the other hand, have the potential to be more engaging than music alone. When we listen to a book while exercising, we might get completely immersed in the plot, making the time fly by. Furthermore, audiobooks may provide cerebral exercise and a physical workout since we must follow the storyline and recall elements from prior chapters.

It's critical to choose music or an audiobook to listen to during a workout that corresponds to the intensity of the activity. Upbeat and fast-paced music, for example, may be more suited for aerobic exercises, while slower, more soothing music may be better suited for yoga or stretching.

When choosing music or audiobooks, one must consider personal tastes. Choosing something we appreciate and are comfortable with may assist in improving and enriching the whole experience.

Listening to music or audiobooks while exercising may have mental health advantages and make exercises more pleasurable. Music has been found in studies to improve mood and lessen symptoms of anxiety and despair. Similarly, audiobooks may give escape and relaxation, which can be helpful to one's mental health.

In conclusion, listening to music or an audiobook while working out may bring a variety of advantages. It may improve performance by elevating mood, decreasing perceived effort, making the experience more pleasurable, and bringing mental health advantages. It is important to consider personal tastes and the intensity of the workout when choosing what to listen to. Incorporating this approach into our training regimen may help to make exercise a more joyful and long-lasting habit.

71. TAKING BREAKS DURING THE WORKDAY TO STAND UP, STRETCH, OR MOVE AROUND

It is normal in today's environment to spend lengthy periods sitting at a desk or in front of a computer screen. This sedentary lifestyle may harm our physical and mental health by raising the risk of obesity, diabetes, and cardiovascular disease, as well as causing back pain, neck discomfort, and headaches. Taking frequent pauses throughout the workplace to get up, stretch, or move about, on the other hand, may have considerable health and productivity advantages.

Taking brief breaks every hour has been demonstrated in studies to enhance overall job performance, raise energy levels, and lower the risk of musculoskeletal diseases. Standing up and moving about for a few minutes may assist in relieving muscle and joint stress, enhance blood flow to the brain, and lower the risk of eye strain and headaches. Taking breaks has also been demonstrated to lower stress and increase mental wellness, resulting in higher work satisfaction and overall quality of life.

Setting a timer or scheduling reminders to take a break every hour is an easy method to include breaks in your workweek. During these pauses, try to get up, stretch, and walk about for a few minutes. This may be going for a little stroll around the office, stretching lightly, or just getting up and moving your arms and legs. Pausing to get a drink or a glass of water or a nutritious snack may also help you keep hydrated and fed throughout the day.

It's vital to remember that breaks should be taken in addition to, not instead of, regular exercise. While brief vacations may benefit both physical and mental health, they do not replace regular physical exercise. Walking, running, swimming, or cycling for at least 30 minutes most days of the week is recommended by experts. Frequent exercise combined with frequent breaks throughout the workplace may assist in preventing the harmful effects of sedentary behavior and enhance overall health and well-being.

Standing up, stretching, or moving about throughout the working may have considerable advantages for our physical and mental health, as well as our productivity and job happiness. Setting reminders to take a break every hour, getting up and moving about for a few minutes, and remaining hydrated and fed throughout the day may help you incorporate brief breaks into your work routine. While breaks are necessary, they should not be used in place of regular exercise, which should be part of your daily routine. You may alter your life and experience the advantages of a healthier, more active lifestyle by simply adjusting your work habits and prioritizing your health and wellness.

72. USING A STANDING DESK TO REDUCE SEDENTARY TIME

Long-term sitting has been linked to several health issues, including obesity, heart disease, and type 2 diabetes, according to research. Many individuals turn to standing desks to minimize sedentary time and enhance their general health to offset these detrimental consequences.

A standing desk is intended to be used while standing rather than sitting. Standing desks come in various styles, ranging from basic risers that can be put on top of a standard desk to full-sized standing desks that can be adjusted to various heights. Some standing workstations have built-in amenities such as treadmills or cycle pedals, enabling users to exercise while working.

One of the most significant advantages of utilizing a standing desk is that it may assist in minimizing inactive time. When Sitting for an extended amount of time, your body burns fewer calories, and your blood flow decreases, which may contribute to various health issues. You may raise your energy expenditure and enhance your blood flow by standing instead of sitting, lowering your chance of developing health issues connected with sedentary behavior.

Another advantage of a standing desk is that it might help you enhance your posture. When you sit for extended periods, it is simple to acquire bad posture over time, which may contribute to neck and back discomfort. Standing rather than sitting engages your core muscles and promotes improved posture, which may help relieve pain and discomfort.

Using a standing desk may boost your happiness and productivity. Studies have demonstrated that standing raises energy levels and mood, which may translate to better productivity and attention at work. You can also prevent the afternoon slump many individuals suffer after sitting for hours if you reduce your inactive time.

While there are several advantages to utilizing a standing desk, it is critical to utilize it correctly to prevent any bad consequences. Standing for an extended period may cause leg and foot discomfort. Therefore, taking breaks and alternating between standing and sitting during the day is important. It is also critical to have an ergonomically built standing workstation to guarantee good posture and limit the chance of damage.

Utilizing a standing desk may help you minimize inactive time and enhance your overall health. You may be able to improve your posture, minimize your chance of developing health issues related to sedentary behavior, and raise your energy and productivity levels by adding a standing desk to your work routine.

73. PRACTICING GOOD POSTURE TO REDUCE BACK PAIN AND IMPROVE BREATHING

Good posture is a sometimes ignored part of general health and well-being. Poor posture may cause various medical problems, including back pain, neck discomfort, migraines, and decreased lung function. Good posture, on the other hand, may enhance your general physical function and help you avoid pain and suffering.

Reduced back discomfort is one of the primary advantages of proper posture. Poor posture may put tension on the back muscles and ligaments, causing pain and even damage over time. In contrast, proper posture may assist in uniformly distributing the body's weight, minimizing strain and tension in the back muscles. This may help you avoid persistent back discomfort while increasing your mobility and flexibility.

Aside from relieving back discomfort, excellent posture may help with breathing and lung function. When you slump or bend over, your chest cavity gets squeezed, making deep breathing more difficult. This may lead to exhaustion, shortness of breath, and other respiratory issues. You may open up your chest and allow for more effective breathing by keeping proper posture and sitting or standing up straight. This may boost your energy, decrease stress, and enhance your physical and mental well-being.

You may take various basic measures throughout the day to cultivate proper posture. Sit with your feet flat on the floor, your back straight, your shoulders relaxed, and your head erect. Crossing your legs or sitting in the same posture for extended periods may lead to stiffness and pain. Stand with your weight equally distributed between both feet and avoid locking your knees or slouching forward. To support your posture, maintain a neutral spine and activate your core muscles.

Taking pauses during the day to stretch and move about might also be beneficial. This may assist in reducing stiffness and soreness while also promoting excellent circulation. Gentle exercise, such as yoga or Pilates, may also help improve posture and alleviate back discomfort.

In conclusion, excellent posture is crucial to general health and well-being. You may relieve discomfort, enhance breathing and lung function, and improve your overall physical and mental health by keeping excellent posture. Simple efforts like sitting up straight and activating your core muscles throughout the day will help improve posture and avoid pain and discomfort in the long run.

74. TAKING BREAKS FROM THE SCREEN TO REST YOUR EYES AND PREVENT HEADACHES

It takes a lot of work to avoid screens in today's environment. We are always surrounded by technology that generates blue light and strains our eyes, from cell phones to computers to televisions. Consequently, it is important to take pauses from screen time to relax your eyes and avoid headaches.

Prolonged computer time has been linked to digital eye strain, a disease characterized by dry, itchy eyes, impaired vision, headaches, and neck and shoulder discomfort. Screen blue light may interrupt our circadian clock, causing sleep difficulties and weariness. Furthermore, gazing at screens for long periods may create eye tiredness, making it difficult to concentrate on activities and decreasing productivity.

The 20-20-20 rule is one approach to avoid digital eye strain. Take a 20-second break from your screen every 20 minutes and gaze at an item 20 feet away for 20 seconds. This practice may aid in the relaxation of your eye muscles and the reduction of weariness. Furthermore, it is critical to blink often while using screens since gazing at displays might induce us to blink less frequently, resulting in dry eyes.

Adjusting the lighting at your office is another approach to prevent eye strain. Position your computer screen to reduce glare and reflection, and adjust the brightness and contrast to your liking. You may also purchase an anti-glare screen or a blue light filter to limit the quantity of blue light produced by your screen.

It's also critical to take breaks from screen usage regularly. Take a break from your computer or phone every hour and do something that doesn't require displays. Take a quick stroll, stretch, or perform some exercises to relieve eye strain and enhance circulation throughout your body.

Incorporating mindfulness and relaxation practices into your daily routine may also aid in the reduction of digital eye strain. Meditation, deep breathing, and yoga may all assist in decreasing stress and enhance general well-being, which can help improve eye health.

Finally, getting adequate sleep is critical for maintaining eye health. Blue light from displays may alter our sleep habits, making falling and remaining asleep more difficult. To reduce the influence of screens on your sleep, avoid using them for at least an hour before going to bed, and keep your bedroom dark and silent. In addition, for general health and well-being, aim for 7-9 hours of sleep every night.

In conclusion, regular breaks from screen time are critical for both eye health and general well-being. Adhering to the 20-20-20 rule, changing lighting, you may lessen digital eye strain and headaches by changing your screen settings, taking frequent breaks, and adding mindfulness and relaxation practices into your daily routine. Prioritizing sleep may also reduce the influence of screens on your sleep patterns and enhance overall health. So, take care of your eyes and give them the rest they need to work properly.

75. DO MENTAL EXERCISES LIKE CROSSWORD PUZZLES OR SUDOKU, TO KEEP YOUR BRAIN SHARP.

Mental activities such as crossword puzzles and Sudoku have become popular as individuals seek techniques to preserve cognitive function and avoid age-related deterioration. While mental exercises cannot promise that they can prevent cognitive decline or dementia, studies have shown that they may aid in increasing memory and processing speed.

Researchers at the University of California, Berkeley discovered that cognitively challenging activities such as crossword puzzles and Sudoku might aid in boosting cognitive function and guard against memory impairment in older persons. Over 2,000 individuals aged 18 to 95 were invited to complete a battery of cognitive tests and report on their participation in cognitively demanding activities. The researchers discovered that people who participated in more cognitively challenging activities had superior cognitive function and were less likely to suffer from memory impairment.

Other research has shown that participating in mental exercises may assist individuals of all ages to enhance their cognitive performance. For example, research published in the journal Neurology discovered that participating in cognitively challenging activities may help lower the risk of cognitive deterioration in older persons. The investigation included Over 1100 people aged 75 to 85 who were tracked for up to seven years. The researchers discovered that people who participated in cognitively stimulating activities had a 63% lower chance of cognitive deterioration than those who did not.

But what is it about mental workouts that might aid in cognitive function improvement? Mental exercises, according to experts, serve to boost cognitive performance by activating the brain and fostering the formation of new neural connections. We challenge our brains to think in new and unusual ways when we do mental exercises, which may enhance memory, processing speed, and general cognitive performance.

There are many more mental workouts than crossword puzzles and Sudoku that might assist in keeping the brain sharp. Learning a new ability, such as playing an instrument or speaking a new language, may be an excellent method to stimulate the brain and encourage the formation of new neural connections. Reading, writing, and participating in social activities may aid in keeping the brain busy and boost cognitive performance.

While participating in mental exercises might benefit cognitive function, it is not a guarantee against cognitive decline or dementia. Other variables, such as genetics and lifestyle, influence cognitive performance and dementia risk. Conversely, engaging in cognitively stimulating tasks may be a useful tool for enhancing general brain health and sustaining cognitive function.

In conclusion, mental activities such as crossword puzzles and Sudoku may aid in keeping the brain sharp and boost cognitive performance. According to research, participating in cognitively challenging activities may help lower the risk of cognitive and memory loss and encourage the formation of new neural connections in the brain. While mental exercises cannot prevent cognitive decline, they may be an effective strategy for preserving cognitive function and increasing general brain health.

76. EXPANDING YOUR KNOWLEDGE AND KEEPING YOUR MIND ACTIVE BY READING BOOKS OR ARTICLES

Reading is a very beneficial activity that may boost your intellect and general health in various ways. Whether you like to read books or articles, it is important to include reading into your daily routine. In this part, we'll look at the advantages of reading and give you some pointers on incorporating it into your life.

To begin with, reading is a wonderful approach to broaden your knowledge and discover new things. You may develop a better grasp of the world around you by reading books or articles on subjects that interest you. This may help you learn new skills, extend your horizons, and sharpen your critical thinking abilities. Reading also increases your imagination and creativity, which can be beneficial in various situations.

Another advantage of reading is that it keeps your mind engaged and healthy. Just like your body needs exercise to keep healthy, your brain requires stimulation to remain sharp. Reading may give such stimulation, preventing cognitive decline and age-related memory loss. Reading has also been proven to relieve stress and increase mood, making it an excellent method to relax and unwind after a hard day.

You may use several techniques to integrate more reading into your life. Setting up a definite time each day for reading, such as in the morning or before bed, is one option. You can also establish a goal for how many books or articles you want to read in a given time and keep track of your progress. Joining a book club or reading group may also help you remain motivated and interact with others who share your interests.

When deciding what to read, choosing information you love and find intriguing is critical. This might include reading books or articles on interesting themes and experimenting with various genres and writing styles. To keep things fresh, consider switching between fiction and nonfiction or reading works by various writers from different historical periods.

There are several format possibilities to pick from. Some individuals prefer physical books over e-books or audiobooks. Experiment with several formats to determine which one works best for you. Remember that audiobooks might be an excellent choice for individuals short on time or struggling to concentrate on printed information.

In conclusion, reading is a wonderful habit to develop for many reasons. It may help you learn more, keep your mind busy and healthy, decrease stress, and enhance your mood. Create a specified time each day for reading, create goals, or integrate more reading into your life. Remember to choose stuff you appreciate and find intriguing, and experiment with various forms to determine what works best for you.

77. TRYING NEW HOBBIES OR ACTIVITIES TO PUSH YOURSELF AND LEARN NEW SKILLS

Trying new hobbies or activities may be a fun and productive way to push yourself, broaden your skill set, and improve your general well-being. Participating in new and different activities may bring success and pleasure while encouraging cognitive and emotional development. Engaging in new activities has been demonstrated in studies to increase mental health, cognitive performance, and overall life satisfaction (Marmeleira, Garrido, & Marques, 2013).

Focusing on things you've always wanted to attempt but haven't been able to do is one technique to explore new hobbies or interests. This might range from learning a new language or musical instrument to participating in a new sport or physical activity. Consider your interests and ambitions while choosing a new hobby or pastime. Choosing something you love that corresponds to your beliefs and tastes is important.

Experimenting with new interests or activities may also be a fantastic way to meet new people and broaden your social network. This is particularly crucial for those who feel alienated or detached from others. Joining a club or organization focused on a certain hobby or interest may give a feeling of connection and community, while chances to learn from others and exchange experiences are provided.

Trying new hobbies or activities may enhance cognitive and emotional development and social advantages. It has been shown that engaging in new situations improves cognitive performance, particularly memory and executive function (Leung & Zhong, 2017). This is likely owing to the fact that new experiences force the brain to work harder, creating new neural connections and driving brain cell development. Trying new things also fosters emotional development by introducing people to new viewpoints and experiences, which can extend their knowledge of the world and their role in it.

Finally, engaging in new hobbies or activities may bring a feeling of achievement and personal development. Learning a new skill or attaining a personal goal may boost self-efficacy and confidence, which can carry over into other aspects of life. This also gives you a feeling of purpose and meaning, a crucial component of overall happiness.

In conclusion, exploring new hobbies or activities may be a fun and productive way to push yourself, broaden your skill set, and improve your general well-being. Learning a new language, attempting a new sport, or picking up a new activity brings excitement and success while fostering cognitive and emotional development. You may enjoy the advantages of trying new things by picking activities that coincide with your interests and aspirations.

78. DOING DEEP BREATHING EXERCISES TO REDUCE STRESS AND ANXIETY

Deep breathing exercises have been demonstrated to be an excellent stress and anxiety reduction strategy. Because these exercises may be done anywhere and at any time, they are a handy and accessible technique to improve daily relaxation and peace. In this part, we'll look at the advantages of deep breathing, how to perform them, and how to incorporate them into your daily routine.

Deep breathing exercises can stimulate the body's relaxation response, one of its key advantages. Our sympathetic nervous system triggers the "fight or flight" reaction when we are stressed or apprehensive. This may cause physical symptoms, such as rapid heartbeat, shallow breathing, and muscular tightness. On the other hand, deep breathing exercises stimulate the parasympathetic nerve system, which is in charge of the relaxation response in the body. This may result in a slower heart rate, less muscular tension, and a sensation of peace and relaxation.

Deep breathing exercises come in various forms, but one of the most frequent is diaphragmatic breathing. To begin diaphragmatic breathing, sit comfortably with your feet flat on the ground and your hands resting on your lap. Close your eyes or lessen your sight and focus on your breathing. Inhale deeply through your nose, filling your lungs and expanding your belly. Hold your breath for a time, then gently exhale through your lips, allowing your tummy to contract as you let go of the air. Repeat for many breaths, concentrating on the feeling of the breath traveling in and out of your body.

Equal breathing is another sort of deep breathing exercise that includes inhaling and exhaling for an equal number of counts. To begin this exercise, choose a comfortable sitting posture with your hands on your lap. Inhale slowly through your nose for four counts, then exhale slowly for four. Repeat for many breaths, concentrating on the feeling of the breath traveling in and out of your body.

If you're feeling especially worried or nervous, it is beneficial to supplement your deep breathing exercise with a visualization or mantra. You may, for example, imagine yourself in a serene and quiet location or repeat a soothing word to yourself while you breathe. Experiment with several strategies to see which ones work best for you.

Deep breathing exercises may be a great approach to alleviate tension and anxiety in your everyday routine. Here are some pointers to help you make it a habit:

1. Make time each day to practice deep breathing techniques. Even a few minutes may have a significant effect.
2. Set a time of day for your breathing exercises, such as first thing in the morning or before bed.
3. Make it a regular part of your regimen. Deep breathing exercises, for example, might be done while waiting in line, during your lunch break, or while traveling.
4. Make use of reminders to assist you in remembering to do your breathing exercises. Set an alarm on your phone or attach a sticky note somewhere noticeable.
5. Deep breathing exercises should be practiced in various contexts so that you may utilize them anytime you need to decrease tension or anxiety.

To summarize, deep breathing exercises are a simple and effective stress and anxiety reduction strategy. Deep breathing may assist in lowering heart rate and muscular tension and generate a sensation of peace and relaxation by triggering the body's relaxation response. Deep breathing exercises come in various forms, and including them in your daily routine may be a powerful method to boost general well-being.

79. PRACTICING PROGRESSIVE MUSCLE RELAXATION TO REDUCE TENSION IN THE BODY

Progressive muscle relaxation is a simple yet effective method for lowering tension and fostering relaxation in the body. To decrease overall muscular tension and generate a feeling of calm, this method includes tensing and then releasing each muscle group in the body one at a time.

Progressive muscle relaxation has been demonstrated in studies to be useful in lowering symptoms of anxiety, depression, and other mental health issues. It may also assist with physical tension symptoms, including headaches and muscular soreness.

Begin by locating a quiet, comfortable area to sit or lie down to practice gradual muscle relaxation. Take a few deep breaths to center yourself and concentrate on the present moment.

Begin by tensing your foot muscles and holding for a few seconds before releasing. Take note of the change in feeling between tension and relaxation. Then, tensing and releasing each muscle group, proceed up to your calves, thighs, buttocks, belly, chest, back, shoulders, arms, hands, neck, and face.

As you practice progressive muscle relaxation, concentrate on your bodily sensations and note the distinctions between tension and relaxation. You may include deep breathing or visualization exercises to maximize the relaxing effect.

Remembering progressive muscle relaxation may not be suitable for everyone, especially those suffering from certain medical disorders or traumas, is crucial. Before beginning any new relaxation or fitness regimen, talking with a healthcare practitioner is always wise.

To summarize, progressive muscle relaxation is a simple and effective approach for lowering tension and fostering relaxation in the body. It may be a useful technique for treating anxiety, sadness, and other mental health disorders, as well as physical tension symptoms. Incorporating progressive muscle relaxation into daily self-care practice may aid in improving general well-being and promoting a feeling of serenity and relaxation.

80. TAKING A BATH WITH EPSOM SALT TO SOOTHE SORE MUSCLES AND PROMOTE RELAXATION

Taking an Epsom salt bath is a simple and inexpensive technique to induce relaxation and ease tight muscles. Epsom salt, also known as magnesium sulfate, has been utilized for its medicinal benefits for generations. When dissolved in warm water, Epsom salt may be absorbed through the skin and give various advantages.

The ability of an Epsom salt bath to relieve tight muscles is one of its key advantages. The magnesium in Epsom salt is a natural muscle relaxant that may assist in relieving muscular discomfort and stress. This is especially good after a strong exercise or a long day of physical activity.

Epsom salt, in addition to its muscle-relaxing qualities, may aid in relaxation and stress reduction. Our body temperature increases when we soak in warm water, which may assist in fostering emotions of peace and relaxation. The magnesium in Epsom salt may help to control stress hormones and produce a feeling of relaxation; therefore, adding it to the bath can improve this impact.

To take an Epsom salt bath, fill your bathtub halfway with warm water and add 1-2 cups of Epsom salt, soak in the bath for 20-30 minutes after stirring the water to dissolve the salt. You may add a few drops of essential oils to the bathwater for an extra aromatherapy boost.

It is crucial to highlight that although Epsom salt baths are usually considered safe, certain precautions should be taken. Before using Epsom salt, anyone with specific health concerns, such as diabetes, high blood pressure, or renal difficulties, should see their doctor. Furthermore, staying hydrated is critical when soaking in an Epsom salt bath since the warm water might promote dehydration.

In conclusion, having an Epsom salt bath may be an easy and effective technique to induce relaxation and ease painful muscles. The magnesium in Epsom salt may help relieve muscular pain and stress, while the warm water can encourage sensations of peace and relaxation. While Epsom salt is typically safe, it is vital to see your doctor before using it if you have specific medical concerns and to remain hydrated while soaking in the bath.

81. USING ESSENTIAL OILS FOR AROMATHERAPY OR TO PROMOTE RELAXATION

Aromatherapy or relaxing with essential oils is a natural and growingly popular technique to assist mental and emotional well-being. Aromatherapy uses essential oils, which are concentrated extracts of plants, to enhance physical and psychological well-being. Essential oils are recognized for their relaxing, elevating, and soothing effects and may be utilized in many ways, including inhalation, massage, and diffusion.

The capacity of essential oils to induce relaxation and relieve tension and anxiety is one of its primary advantages. Aromatherapy may help to quiet the mind and relax the body, making it an excellent technique for controlling anxiety and depression symptoms. Lavender, bergamot, and chamomile essential oils are very effective in promoting relaxation and reducing sensations of tension and anxiety.

One of the most frequent methods to utilize essential oils for relaxation is inhalation. Add a few drops of essential oil to a diffuser or humidifier, or place a drop or two on a tissue or rag and inhale deeply. Inhaling essential oils enables the scent to enter the body via the olfactory system, which may activate a relaxation response in the brain and assist in calming the nervous system.

Massage is another excellent technique to relax using essential oils. Essential oils may be used directly on the skin and massaged into the body when mixed with carrier oils such as coconut or almond oil. This may aid in the relief of muscular tension, the improvement of circulation, and the promotion of a sensation of calm and relaxation. Essential oils like peppermint and eucalyptus are especially effective in relieving muscular pain and promoting physical relaxation.

Finally, essential oils enhance relaxation and well-being in several additional ways. For example, adding a few drops of essential oil to a warm bath may produce a peaceful and pleasant atmosphere. Similarly, applying essential oils in a room spray or on bedding may aid in the creation of a tranquil and restful environment that encourages relaxation and a good night's sleep.

While essential oils are usually considered safe, they should be used with care and under the supervision of a skilled practitioner. Because essential oils are very concentrated, they should always be diluted before use. Additionally, certain oils may cause skin irritation or allergic responses in some persons. Furthermore, many essential oils may be unsafe to use during pregnancy or for people with specific medical problems.

To summarize, aromatherapy using essential oils is a natural and effective technique to induce relaxation and relieve tension and anxiety. Essential oils, whether utilized via inhalation, massage, or other means, may assist in quieting the mind and body and create a relaxing environment. To ensure safe and effective usage, essential oils should be used with care and under the supervision of a skilled practitioner.

82. GETTING A MASSAGE OR ACUPUNCTURE TO PROMOTE RELAXATION AND REDUCE PAIN

Massage therapy and acupuncture have recently become popular to promote relaxation, reduce pain, and improve general health. Both rituals have ancient origins and have been employed for millennia in many societies worldwide. In this part, we'll look at the advantages of massage treatment and acupuncture and how they might fit into a healthy lifestyle.

Massage therapy uses pressure, movement, and tension to manipulate soft tissues, such as muscles, tendons, and ligaments. A qualified massage therapist usually administers it, and it may be personalized to the requirements and preferences of the individual. Massage treatment has been found to provide a variety of advantages, including the promotion of relaxation, the reduction of stress and anxiety, the improvement of circulation, and the reduction of muscular tension and discomfort.

Massage therapy's capacity to induce relaxation and alleviate stress is one of its key advantages. Endorphins, the body's natural painkillers and mood lifters, are released when soft tissues are physically manipulated. This may result in a state of profound relaxation and peacefulness, which can aid in the reduction of stress and anxiety.

Massage treatment has also been demonstrated to help with circulation. Massage stroke pressure and movement may assist in enhancing blood flow and oxygenation to muscles and other tissues, improving general health and lowering the risk of certain illnesses, including heart disease and stroke.

Massage treatment, in addition to inducing relaxation and boosting circulation, may be useful in relieving muscular tension and discomfort. Massage strokes with pressure and movement may assist the release of knots and adhesions in the muscles, which can cause pain and suffering. Massage treatment may be especially beneficial for chronic pain problems such as arthritis or fibromyalgia.

Acupuncture is another ancient treatment used to enhance health and well-being for ages. It involves inserting small needles into certain places on the body to balance the flow of energy or qi throughout the body. Acupuncture has been demonstrated to provide a variety of advantages, including pain relief, improved sleep, and stress and anxiety reduction.

One of the most important advantages of acupuncture is its capacity to relieve pain. The insertion of the needles may cause endorphin release, which can relieve pain and increase relaxation. Acupuncture has been demonstrated to be very useful in the treatment of chronic pain disorders such as back pain, neck pain, and headaches.

Acupuncture may also help you sleep better. Many people who get acupuncture report better sleep quality and duration, which may have various health advantages. Improved sleep may improve moods, energy, and general health and well-being.

Finally, studies have indicated that acupuncture may help with tension and anxiety. Acupuncture may induce relaxation and alleviate symptoms of stress and anxiety. This may have various beneficial consequences on one's general health and well-being.

In conclusion, massage therapy and acupuncture are two techniques that may be implemented into a healthy lifestyle to promote relaxation, pain relief, and general health and well-being. Both rituals have ancient origins and have been employed for millennia in many societies worldwide. To attempt massage therapy or acupuncture, consult a professional practitioner about your specific requirements and preferences. You may enjoy a variety of health advantages and enhance your overall quality of life by implementing these activities into your life.

83. PRACTICING VISUALIZATION OR GUIDED MEDITATION TO REDUCE STRESS AND IMPROVE FOCUS

Visualization or guided meditation is an effective stress-reduction and focus-improvement practice. Visualization is a mental method that includes envisioning a tranquil or happy scene to induce relaxation. Guided meditation, on the other hand, is listening to an audio track that guides you through focusing on your breath and thoughts.

Numerous studies have demonstrated that visualization and guided meditation improve mental health by lowering anxiety and sadness and increasing general well-being. This is because these approaches enable you to concentrate on happy thoughts and feelings while also assisting you in releasing negative emotions and tension.

According to one study done by Stanford University researchers, visualization and guided meditation increased cognitive function in students. Participants who listened to a guided meditation audio recording significantly improved their working memory, attention span, and general cognitive performance. According to the findings of this research, visualization and guided meditation may be effective strategies for increasing attention and productivity.

Furthermore, visualization and guided meditation have been shown to reduce stress and anxiety levels. Researchers at the University of California, San Francisco, discovered that mindfulness meditation, which includes focused breathing and visualization methods, lowered stress levels in individuals by up to 40%. Similarly, the National Institutes of Health discovered that visualization and guided meditation lowered anxiety symptoms in cancer patients.

Including visualization and guided meditation in your daily routine helps you sleep better. Studies have demonstrated meditation to help you fall asleep quicker and remain asleep longer. This is because meditation may assist you in relaxing and releasing unwanted thoughts and emotions that may keep you awake.

Find a quiet and comfortable spot to sit or lie down without interruptions to practice visualization or guided meditation. You may either listen to an audio-guided meditation track or shut your eyes and envision a tranquil or happy environment. Concentrate on your breathing and attempt to release any unpleasant ideas or feelings.

You may also attempt progressive muscle relaxation, which is tensing and then relaxing each muscle group in your body one at a time while picturing a tranquil or good situation. This practice might help you calm your thoughts and alleviate bodily stress.

In conclusion, practicing visualization or guided meditation may have significant mental and physical health advantages. It may aid in the reduction of stress and anxiety, the enhancement of cognitive function and attention, and the enhancement of sleep quality. Incorporating these tactics into your everyday routine will help you live a happier and more serene life.

84. SETTING ASIDE TIME EACH DAY FOR SELF-REFLECTION OR JOURNALING

Getting caught up in the rush and bustle of everyday living in today's fast-paced world is easy. On the other hand, taking a few minutes each day for self-reflection or writing may be a powerful approach to decreasing stress, developing clarity, and enhancing general well-being.

Self-reflection entails pausing from our regular routines to examine our thoughts, emotions, and behaviors. By doing so, we may obtain a greater knowledge of ourselves, our motives, and our values. As a result, we may make better judgments and live more rewarding lives.

Journaling is one method of self-reflection. We may uncover patterns in our thinking and behavior by writing down our ideas and emotions. It may also be used for problem-solving and goal planning. We may monitor our improvement over time and achieve a stronger self-awareness by maintaining a notebook.

Self-reflection and writing have been demonstrated in studies to offer a variety of advantages for our mental health and well-being. Research published in the journal Advances in Psychiatric Treatment, for example, discovered that reflective writing may be an effective strategy to lessen depression and anxiety symptoms.

Another study published in the Journal of Psychosocial Oncology discovered that journaling may enhance cancer patients' quality of life by lowering symptoms of sadness and anxiety and increasing emotions of well-being.

Self-reflection and writing offer physical health advantages in addition to mental health benefits. According to research published in the Journal of Psychosomatic Research, expressive writing (journaling) may boost immune system functioning and lessen disease symptoms in people with chronic illnesses.

So, how can we include self-reflection and writing into our everyday lives? One easy technique is setting aside a few minutes each day to focus on our thoughts and emotions. This might be journaling or just spending a few quiet minutes to contemplate.

Another alternative is to direct our self-reflection using suggestions or questions. For instance, we may question ourselves:

What do I have reason to be thankful for today?

What obstacles did I meet today, and how did I overcome them?

What should I do to be more satisfied in life?

By responding to these questions, we may obtain a better understanding of our ideas and emotions, as well as discover opportunities for development and progress.

In conclusion, self-reflection and writing effectively enhance mental and physical health. We may achieve more self-awareness and make more informed judgments by spending a few minutes each day to focus on our thoughts and emotions. Finding time for oneself, whether via writing, meditation, or other types of self-reflection, is crucial for living a healthy and fulfilled life.

85. PRACTICING GRATITUDE AND FOCUSING ON THE POSITIVE ASPECTS OF YOUR LIFE

Gratitude is recognizing and appreciating the good things in our lives, large and small. Gratitude practice has been proven to improve our mental health, relationships, and general well-being. According to studies, practicing thankfulness may lead to higher happiness, better sleep, less stress and anxiety, and even better physical health.

Keeping a gratitude diary, where you write down things you are grateful for daily, is one approach to practicing thankfulness. This may assist you in focusing on the good parts of your life and developing a more optimistic outlook. Another approach to practicing gratitude is communicating it to others, whether via a genuine thank you message, a kind gift, or just telling someone how much you appreciate them.

It is also crucial to concentrate on the good parts of your life in addition to practicing appreciation. It's easy to get caught up in negative thinking and difficulties, but research shows that concentrating on the good may significantly influence our well-being. When concentrating on the good, we create a more optimistic mindset and enjoy better pleasure and well-being.

Engaging in positive self-talk is one approach to concentrating on the good. This entails turning negative ideas into good ones. Instead of thinking, "I'll never be able to do this," consider, "I may not be able to do this right now, but with practice and effort, I can improve." Engaging in things that offer pleasure and contentment is another approach to concentrating on the good. This might be anything from spending time with family and friends to participating in a hobby or helping in your community.

It's vital to remember that being grateful and concentrating on the good elements of our lives does not imply dismissing or rejecting the problems and difficulties we experience. Rather, it entails confronting these difficulties more optimistically and appreciating the wonderful parts of our lives alongside the challenging ones.

In conclusion, concentrating on the good parts of our lives and practicing thankfulness may influence our well-being. We may boost our happiness, strengthen our relationships, and improve our physical health by creating more positive thinking and participating in things that offer us pleasure and satisfaction. So, each day, take a minute to think about what you are grateful for, communicate your gratitude to others, and concentrate on the good elements of your life. Your health will appreciate it.

86. SEEKING HELP FROM A THERAPIST OR COUNSELOR WHEN NECESSARY

Seeking help from a therapist or counselor when required may be a significant tool in improving your life. While changing your lifestyle might be difficult, having someone to speak to about your challenges and triumphs can help keep you on track.

Therapists and counselors are skilled experts who may provide advice and assistance in dealing with a variety of concerns, such as stress, anxiety, despair, and addiction. They may assist you in identifying the root causes of bad behaviors and developing ways to overcome them.

One advantage of obtaining help from a therapist or counselor is that they give you a secure and private environment to examine your ideas and emotions. They may assist you in developing coping methods to deal with stress and anxiety, which can frequently lead to undesirable habits like binge eating or drug addiction.

Working with a therapist or counselor also has the added benefit of providing accountability and encouragement. Setting goals and measuring progress with the assistance of a professional may help you remain motivated and dedicated to your healthy habits.

It is important to understand that getting help from a therapist or counselor is not a show of weakness but rather a proactive move toward bettering your mental and emotional health. Getting expert care for mental health difficulties is just as important as getting medical attention for a physical disease.

There are a few things to consider before seeking the help of a therapist or counselor. First and foremost, you must locate someone who is a good match for you. Look for a therapist or counselor specializing in the issues you're dealing with and with whom you feel comfortable discussing.

Second, communicate openly and honestly with your therapist or counselor. The more they understand your ideas, emotions, and habits, the more prepared they will be to assist you in developing successful transformation tactics.

Third, it is critical to be patient and dedicated to the process. Working with a therapist or counselor to make lifestyle changes takes time. However, with commitment and perseverance, the rewards of obtaining expert assistance may be life-changing.

In conclusion, receiving help from a therapist or counselor may be extremely beneficial in improving your life with good practices. Working with a professional may help you overcome the obstacles by giving you a safe and private environment to examine your ideas and emotions, as well as accountability and encouragement.

Identify the root causes of harmful behaviors and devise effective transformation tactics. If you're thinking about obtaining professional help, make sure you locate someone who is a good match for you, that you're open and honest with them, and that you're patient and devoted to the process.

87. PRACTICING FORGIVENESS AND LETTING GO OF GRUDGES

Forgiveness is a strong technique for overcoming emotions of rage, wrath, and bitterness. Holding grudges may cause bad feelings, stress, and even physical health concerns, but practicing forgiveness can enhance our mental and physical health. This part will review the significance of practicing forgiveness and letting go of grudges.

To begin, it is critical to understand what forgiving entails. Forgiveness does not imply forgetting or tolerating wrongdoing. It is about admitting the hurt and letting go of the anger and resentment that might keep us rooted in the past. Forgiveness is difficult and often involves a concerted effort to shift our ideas and feelings.

One of the advantages of forgiving is that it might boost our mental health. Forgiving others has been found in studies to reduce symptoms of despair and anxiety while increasing sentiments of optimism and hope. Forgiveness also helps us to let go of bad feelings and concentrate on good interactions, which may help us create stronger connections with others.

Forgiveness, in addition to enhancing our emotional wellness, may offer physical health advantages. Chronic anger and resentment may raise stress hormone levels in the body, hurting the cardiovascular and immunological systems. We may decrease these harmful consequences on our physical health by letting go of grudges and practicing forgiveness.

So, how do we go about practicing forgiveness? Here are some pointers:

1. Recognize the hurt that has been inflicted. Acknowledging the harm done rather than attempting to downplay or deny it is critical.
2. Choose to let go of your bitterness and fury. This might be challenging, but it is a necessary step in forgiving.
3. Empathy should be practiced. Try to grasp the other person's motives and intentions by seeing things from their point of view.
4. Express your emotions. Talk to the injured individual and communicate your thoughts calmly and courteously, if appropriate.
5. Practice forgiving yourself. To go on and make meaningful changes in our lives, we must forgive ourselves for previous errors and failings.

Practicing forgiveness and letting go of grudges may have significant mental and physical health advantages. It can enhance interpersonal connections, decrease stress, and boost general well-being. While it is not easy to forgive, it is a talent that can be learned and practiced over time. We may alter our lives and create a better future by letting go of our anger and resentment.

88. CONNECTING WITH OTHERS THROUGH VOLUNTEERING OR COMMUNITY SERVICE

Volunteering, often known as community service, is donating your time, talents, or resources to assist others in your community. This is a fantastic opportunity to interact with people while developing a feeling of purpose and satisfaction. Volunteering has several advantages, including personal development, enhanced mental health, and a deeper feeling of community.

Personal development is one of the key advantages of volunteering. Volunteering allows you to gain new skills, enhance your talents, and push yourself in new ways. Volunteering might also assist you in gaining perspective on your life and appreciating what you have. It may be an excellent way to go out of your comfort zone and try something new, which can be powerful and confidence-building.

Another advantage of volunteering is that it improves one's mental health. Helping others gives you a feeling of purpose and satisfaction, which may improve your mood and decrease stress. Volunteering has been demonstrated to boost general well-being and minimize symptoms of despair and anxiety. It also helps you feel more connected to your community and less lonely and isolated.

Finally, volunteering is a great method to strengthen your feeling of community. You may help others by volunteering. Meet new people and form bonds with those who share your beliefs and interests. This may result in new friendships and a stronger feeling of belonging. Volunteering gives you the sense that you're making a difference in your community, which can be powerful and motivating.

There are several possibilities for volunteering and community service if you are interested. You may assist needy individuals by volunteering at a local nonprofit organization, participating in community clean-up activities, or offering your talents. The goal is to select an opportunity that corresponds to your interests and values so that you can make the most of your experience.

In conclusion, volunteering or community service is a great way to connect with people while developing a feeling of purpose and satisfaction. It provides several advantages, including personal development, enhanced mental health, and a deeper feeling of community. If you want to volunteer, several options are available; the key is to select one that matches your interests and beliefs. You may make a difference in your community and life by volunteering your time, talents, or resources to assist others.

89. AVOIDING NEGATIVE SELF-TALK AND PRACTICALLY IMPLEMENTING SELF-COMPASSION

The mental conversation that occurs in our brains is referred to as self-talk. It tremendously influences our mental well-being and may be beneficial or bad. Criticizing oneself, dwelling on perceived defects or inadequacies, and using harsh words are all examples of negative self-talk. Positive self-talk, on the other hand, entails encouraging oneself, concentrating on one's abilities, and using sympathetic words.

According to research, negative self-talk may raise tension, anxiety, and depression, but good self-talk can boost self-esteem, confidence, and general well-being. Avoiding negative self-talk and practicing self-compassion may, therefore, significantly influence our mental health.

Self-compassion entails treating oneself with care, understanding, and acceptance, even when one has failed or fallen short. It is not the same as self-indulgence but rather a technique of connecting with and knowing oneself. Individuals may learn to be more forgiving of themselves by practicing self-compassion, which can lead to lower stress and greater emotional well-being.

Positive self-talk is one technique to cultivate self-compassion. This entails using terminology that is; instead of being judgmental and rude, be helpful and nice. Instead of stating, "I'm so stupid," say, "I made a mistake, but I'm still a capable and intelligent person." This form of self-talk may aid in developing a more positive self-image and reducing emotions of self-doubt.

Self-care activities are another approach to cultivating self-compassion. These may include obtaining adequate sleep, eating a good diet, exercising regularly, and participating in hobbies that offer pleasure or relaxation. Individuals may enhance their well-being and lessen stress and worry by attending to their physical and emotional requirements.

Individuals may also cultivate self-compassion via mindfulness activities. Paying attention to the present moment with nonjudgmental awareness is what mindfulness entails. Individuals may benefit from this by being more aware of their thoughts and emotions and learning to observe them without judgment or condemnation. Individuals may learn to be more sympathetic toward themselves and lessen sentiments of self-criticism by practicing this form of awareness.

Finally, remember that self-compassion is a skill that can be learned and improved over time. It takes time and effort, but the rewards may be substantial. Individuals may enhance their mental and emotional well-being and develop a more positive self-image by practicing self-compassion.

In conclusion, negative self-talk may raise tension, anxiety, and depression, but good self-talk can boost self-esteem, confidence, and general well-being. As a result, practicing self-compassion and avoiding negative self-talk may have a significant influence on our mental health. Even in the face of personal mistakes or weaknesses, self-compassion entails treating oneself with respect, understanding, and acceptance. This form of self-talk may aid in developing a more positive self-image and reducing emotions of self-doubt. Self-compassion may also be practiced via self-care, mindfulness techniques, and learning to notice one's thoughts and feelings without judgment or condemnation. Finally, practicing self-compassion is a skill that can be learned and cultivated over time, resulting in better mental and emotional well-being.

90. SETTING BOUNDARIES AND SAYING NO WHEN NECESSARY TO PROTECT YOUR TIME AND ENERGY

It is natural to feel overwhelmed and overworked in today's fast-paced society. Many individuals struggle to make time and energy to follow their goals and interests, much alone care for their physical and mental health. To safeguard your time and energy in such a situation, creating boundaries and learning to say no when required is critical.

Setting boundaries entails identifying, discussing, and adhering to your limitations. Saying no to jobs or activities that do not line with your goals, scheduling time for self-care, and limiting your time spent on social media or other distractions are all examples of this. Setting limits may help you minimize stress and make more room for the things that are important.

Saying no may be challenging, particularly if you prefer to please people or fear losing chances. On the other hand, learning to say no may be powerful and help you concentrate on what is important. It's vital to remember that saying no does not indicate being nasty or selfish; it just means you're looking after yourself and your own needs.

You must first understand your beliefs and priorities to effectively create limits and say no when required. What are the most important things to you? What are your long-term ambitions and goals? You can better focus your time and energy and make choices that match your goals if you understand your values and priorities.

It is also critical to express your limits clearly and assertively. Setting limitations on your availability, saying no to requests that do not line with your goals, and learning to delegate responsibilities to others when required may all contribute to this. When establishing your limits, being courteous but strong and avoiding apologizing or explaining too much is crucial.

Setting boundaries and saying no is crucial, but so is prioritizing self-care and making time for things that feed your physical and emotional well-being. This might involve physical activity, meditation, time spent in nature, or just relaxing and recharging. Prioritizing self-care may help you decrease stress and enhance your general well-being, allowing you to be more productive and focused on your other hobbies.

In conclusion, learning to establish boundaries and say no when required is crucial to caring for your physical and mental health, decreasing stress, and accomplishing your goals. You can make more room for what matters by knowing your values and goals, clearly and assertively stating your boundaries, and prioritizing self-care.

91. USING A PLANNER OR JOURNAL TO STAY ORGANIZED AND ON TRACK WITH GOALS

Maintaining organization and staying on track with goals is critical to a healthy and productive life. With our hectic schedules and various distractions, remaining focused and working towards our goals may be difficult. Using a planner or diary to help keep us organized and on track is one of the most effective strategies to combat this difficulty.

A planner or diary may be used to record appointments, deadlines, and key events and to define and track goals. It may also be used to record daily routines, habits, and other critical information that might assist us in making good life changes.

Choosing a planner or diary that meets your requirements and tastes is critical. Some individuals prefer a paper-based planner, while others prefer a digital planner. Choosing a calendar or diary that is simple to use and matches your lifestyle is also important.

Once you've decided on a planner or diary, you must utilize it consistently and regularly. This helps you develop the habit of remaining organized and on track with your goals. It also keeps you motivated and focused by allowing you to track your progress toward your goals over time.

Besides keeping a planner or notebook, other tactics may help you remain organized and on track with your goals. Breaking big goals into smaller, more achievable activities is effective. This might make you feel less stressed and more determined to achieve your goals.

Another approach is to prioritize activities according to their significance and urgency. This allows you to concentrate on the most critical activities while avoiding spending time on less important ones. It helps you better organize your time and minimize stress and worry.

Finally, it is critical to be adaptable and flexible in changing situations. Because life is unpredictable, it is critical to be prepared to change your plans and goals as required. You can better manage your time, focus on your goals, and ultimately have a happier and more rewarding life if you stay organized and adaptable.

Keeping a planner or notebook helps you remain organized and on track with your goals. You may overcome the hurdles of contemporary life and accomplish your goals by utilizing a planner or notebook regularly, breaking down big goals into smaller tasks, prioritizing work, and being flexible. Anyone may utilize a planner or diary to alter their life and become the best version of themselves with devotion and effort.

92. GETTING ENOUGH SUNLIGHT TO SUPPORT VITAMIN D PRODUCTION AND IMPROVE MOOD

Getting adequate sunshine is critical for general health and happiness. Sunlight gives us vitamin D necessary for strong bones, a healthy immune system, and mood regulation. Vitamin D advantages are not restricted to physical health; they also play an important part in emotional and psychological well-being. This part will examine how receiving enough sunshine may help with vitamin D production and boost mood.

Vitamin D is a fat-soluble vitamin that the skin produces when exposed to sunshine. It is required to absorb and manage calcium and phosphorus in the body, which is necessary to maintain healthy bones and teeth. Vitamin D also helps the immune system by regulating cell development, decreasing inflammation, and speeding up wound healing.

Vitamin D has a substantial influence on mental health in addition to its physical advantages. Vitamin D insufficiency has been linked to an increased risk of depression, anxiety, and other mood disorders in studies. This is because vitamin D is important for modulating neurotransmitters such as dopamine and serotonin, which are required for mood regulation.

Sunlight exposure is one of the most efficient methods to get vitamin D. When exposed to ultraviolet B (UVB) radiation, which is found in sunshine, the skin manufactures vitamin D. It is crucial to remember, however, that prolonged sun exposure might raise the risk of skin cancer and other skin damage. As a result, striking a balance between obtaining adequate sunshine and protecting the skin from damaging UV radiation is critical.

The quantity of sunshine required to create enough vitamin D varies based on skin tone, geographic location, time of day, and season. For example, people with darker skin tones need more solar exposure to synthesize the same amount of vitamin D as those with lighter skin tones. Similarly, people living closer to the equator get stronger sunshine all year, which might boost vitamin D production.

Instead of depending only on sunshine exposure, the American Academy of Dermatology suggests receiving vitamin D via a mix of diet and supplements. However, sun exposure is crucial for supporting vitamin D production and promoting general health and well-being.

Following a few basic recommendations to maximize the advantages of sunshine exposure while limiting the hazards is important. To begin, try to receive some sunshine exposure early in the morning or late in the afternoon when the sun's rays are less powerful. Second, to protect the skin from damaging UV radiation, wear protective clothes and apply sunscreen with an SPF of at least 30. Finally, aim for 10-15 minutes of sunshine exposure every day, gradually increasing the length over time.

In conclusion, obtaining adequate sunshine is critical for general health and well-being. Sunlight is the major source of vitamin D, which is required for strong bones, a robust immune system, and mood regulation. However, a balance between obtaining adequate sunshine and protecting the skin from damaging UV rays must be struck. It is feasible to receive the numerous advantages of this powerful natural resource by following simple recommendations and integrating sunshine exposure into a healthy lifestyle.

93. SURROUNDING YOURSELF WITH PEOPLE WHO ARE POSITIVE AND SUPPORTIVE

Humans are social beings, and our social interactions and connections shape our lives significantly. Our interactions with others may help or impede our attempts to build and maintain healthy behaviors. This is why it is important to surround ourselves with positive individuals who support our aims and ideals. In this part, we'll look at the advantages of having a supportive social network and provide some advice on how to build one.

The Advantages of a Helpful Social Network

A helpful social network may give our physical and mental well-being several advantages. People with strong social ties live longer, have stronger immunological function, and are less likely to suffer from depression and other mental health disorders, according to research (Cohen et al., 2014; Holt-Lunstad et al., 2010). Furthermore, having supportive friends and family members may help us deal with stress and hardship, essential for our general well-being (Uchino, 2006).

A supportive social network may be a strong incentive for building healthy behaviors. Being in the company of others who share our beliefs and aspirations might help us remain focused and devoted to our health goals. Furthermore, having friends and family members who understand healthy behaviors may give us helpful guidance and support.

Tips for Growing a Positive Social Network

Here are some suggestions for building a helpful social network:

1. Look for people who share your beliefs. Joining an organization or community that shares your interests and beliefs may be an excellent opportunity to meet new individuals who share your aspirations. Finding a group of individuals who share your interests, whether a fitness club, a cooking class, or a volunteer organization, may help you develop a strong and supportive social network.

2. Maintain existing ties. Don't underestimate the influence of your present social network. Try to preserve ties with friends and family members who support your aspirations. Make time for social activities that help you achieve your health goals, such as walking or trying a new healthy food with a friend.

3. Make a good impact. You may have a beneficial influence on others around you just as you benefit from the support

of others. Share your healthy habits and accomplishments with your friends and family, and urge others to join you. You may encourage people to make great changes in their lives by becoming a positive role model.

4. Let go of toxic connections. Unfortunately, not all partnerships are constructive and encouraging. If you have friends or family members who are often negative or critical of you, it may be time to reconsider such ties. Surrounding oneself with negative individuals may be harmful to your health and well-being. Instead, prioritize connections with individuals who encourage and support your endeavors.

5. Make use of technology. Connecting with like-minded people online in today's digital world is simpler than ever. Joining online forums or social media groups relevant to your interests and aspirations may be an excellent way to meet new people and get support.

Summary:

Maintaining our general health and well-being and attaining our health goals requires a supporting social network. We can remain motivated, obtain useful information and guidance, and manage stress and hardship more successfully if we surround ourselves with positive and helpful individuals. We may create a helpful social network by seeking out like-minded persons, nurturing existing ties, being a good influence, letting go of toxic relationships, and using technology.

94. SETTING REALISTIC GOALS AND BREAKING THEM DOWN INTO SMALLER, ACHIEVABLE STEPS

Setting realistic goals is vital to changing your life for the better. A big list of goals and resolutions may easily overwhelm you, leading to emotions of failure and disappointment. However, by breaking down big goals into smaller, more manageable tasks, you may improve your odds of achievement and keep yourself motivated.

Determining what you want to accomplish is the first step in creating realistic goals. Perhaps you want to lose weight, get in shape, or lessen your stress. Your objective must be specific, measurable, achievable, relevant, and time-bound (SMART). This will assist you in remaining focused and tracking your progress along the road.

After you've determined your SMART objective, the following step is to break it down into smaller, more manageable tasks. For example, if you want to lose weight, you may reduce your daily calorie consumption by 500 calories. You can then take it further by planning nutritious foods and snacks, including more physical activity in your daily routine, and keeping a diet and exercise log to monitor your progress.

It is critical to remember that each modest step toward your greater objective is a victory in and of itself. Celebrate your victories along the road to help you remain motivated and on track. Be adaptable and open to changing your goals as required. Life is unpredictable, and unexpected circumstances may lead to setbacks. You can keep moving forward if you are adaptive and ready to adjust.

Enlisting the help of others is another important aspect of developing realistic goals. A support system, whether a friend, family member, or health professional, may help you stay accountable and motivated. It also provides a feeling of camaraderie and support during difficult times.

To summarize, creating realistic goals and breaking them down into smaller, manageable stages is critical to improving your life. You may boost your odds of success and sustain motivation by making your goals SMART, breaking them down into manageable stages, celebrating minor victories, being adaptive, and enlisting the assistance of others.

95. CELEBRATING SMALL SUCCESSES AND ACHIEVEMENTS

Small successes and achievements must be celebrated as part of developing and sustaining good habits. We often fixate on the final goal and fail to recognize the progress we make along the road. We may enhance our enthusiasm, reinforce our good behaviors, and develop resilience to setbacks by recognizing and enjoying minor victories.

One of the major advantages of celebrating small success is the feeling of achievement and joy it brings. It may be intimidating and overwhelming when we set out to do anything. We can, however, generate a feeling of progress and momentum by breaking it down into smaller, more manageable stages. We gain confidence and joy in our successes every time we step ahead.

Furthermore, recognizing little accomplishments keeps us motivated and focused. Recognizing and celebrating our accomplishments strengthens our conviction in ourselves and our capacity to attain our goals. This, in turn, keeps us motivated and committed to our good behaviors. Small triumphs also help to increase accountability. When we share our achievements with others, we develop a feeling of social support and responsibility that may assist us in staying on course.

Another key advantage of celebrating little triumphs is that it helps us develop resilience in adversity. The path to our goals is seldom straightforward, and we are certain to experience obstacles and failures along the way. We may generate positive momentum and a buffer against failures by appreciating our tiny triumphs. Instead of obsessing over setbacks and failures, celebrating minor victories allows us to concentrate on our progress and the good steps we have taken.

There are several methods to commemorate minor wins and successes. Keeping a diary or track of your progress is a simple yet powerful strategy. Whenever you win a tiny triumph or reach a goal, write it down and reflect on the good steps you've achieved. This may be a very effective strategy for reinforcing beneficial behaviors and increasing drive and resilience.

Another method to recognize tiny triumphs is to praise yourself for your efforts. This might be as easy as treating yourself to a favorite food, engaging in an enjoyable hobby or activity, or taking time to rest and recharge. We generate a feeling of positive reinforcement by praising ourselves for our hard work and devotion, which may help us remain motivated and devoted to our healthy habits.

In conclusion, recognizing modest successes and achievements is an important component of developing and sustaining good behaviors. We generate motivation, reinforce beneficial behaviors, and build resilience by noticing and celebrating our success. Small triumphs help us remain focused and dedicated to our goals, whether we maintain a diary, reward ourselves for our hard work, or share our successes with others.

96. AVOIDING PROCRASTINATION AND PRIORITIZING IMPORTANT TASKS

Procrastination is a widespread problem that impacts both personal and professional life. It is the act of delaying or postponing necessary duties, which often results in emotions of guilt, tension, and worry. While procrastination may temporarily relieve the stress of finishing a job, it eventually does more damage than good. Prioritizing critical tasks is a necessary habit that helps people accomplish their goals and enhance their overall quality of life.

Understanding the fundamental causes of procrastination is the first step in overcoming it. Fear of failure, a lack of enthusiasm, and emotions of overload may contribute to procrastination. Individuals may act after identifying the core reason for their procrastination. For example, if a significant contributing component is a fear of failure, people might focus on increasing their self-confidence and establishing more realistic goals.

Individuals may create habits that help them prioritize critical work and address the underlying reasons for procrastination. One successful way is to make a to-do list and prioritize things based on their priority. Individuals may benefit from this. They are focused and driven because they understand what has to be done and can prioritize properly. Setting realistic deadlines for assignments is also crucial since it creates a feeling of urgency and helps people remain on track.

Another beneficial practice is to divide larger activities into smaller, more manageable segments. This may make the process seem less scary and overwhelming as each stage is accomplished, and it can create a feeling of success as each step is completed. It is also critical to provide a suitable atmosphere for work completion. This might include turning off distractions like social media and other technological gadgets and finding a quiet place to concentrate.

Developing effective time management skills may also assist people in prioritizing vital activities. This entails designating specified periods of the day for work completion and avoiding time-wasting diversions during those hours. Setting limits and learning to say no to non-essential jobs or activities helps people remain focused and avoid being overwhelmed.

To summarize, avoiding procrastinating and prioritizing key work are critical habits for success and well-being. Individuals may overcome procrastination and accomplish their goals by recognizing the underlying reasons for procrastination, adopting efficient time management skills, and establishing a favorable atmosphere for task completion. While prioritizing vital tasks may involve work and discipline, the advantages are well worth the effort.

97. TAKING BREAKS WHEN NEEDED TO PREVENT BURNOUT AND INCREASE PRODUCTIVITY

Taking necessary breaks is critical for avoiding burnout and enhancing productivity. Although it may seem paradoxical, taking frequent breaks may increase overall job performance and lead to better results. This part will go over the necessity of taking breaks, how to tell when you need one, and the many sorts of breaks that may be useful.

Burnout is a condition of physical, emotional, and mental depletion produced by lengthy periods of high stress. Burnout may have major consequences for one's general health and well-being, such as an increased risk of depression and anxiety, lower work satisfaction, and decreased productivity. It is critical to detect the signs and symptoms of burnout early on and try to prevent it from worsening.

Taking frequent pauses throughout the day is one of the most efficient methods to avoid burnout. This may involve taking brief breaks every hour or so and larger breaks like lunch or a short stroll outdoors. When you return to work, the key is allowing the mind and body to rest and recharge, which may lead to better attention, concentration, and productivity.

It is also critical to know when a break is required. Feeling fatigued, irritated, and stressed are all symptoms of burnout and weariness. Listen to your body and take breaks when necessary, rather than pushing through and risking greater weariness.

Depending on the person and the scenario, several breaks might be good. Short pauses, such as stretching or taking a brief stroll, help you concentrate and re-energize. Longer breaks, such as taking a lunch break away from work or taking a day off, might be beneficial in dealing with more severe burnout and stress.

Taking breaks that include physical exercise or mindfulness may also be beneficial in reducing burnout and boosting overall wellness. Yoga, meditation, or just going for a stroll outdoors may help to decrease stress and improve emotions of relaxation and serenity.

Taking breaks when required is critical to avoiding burnout and increasing productivity. Recognizing the indications of burnout and weariness and addressing them via frequent breaks and self-care may lead to better overall health and wellness. Listen to your body, pause as required, and participate in activities encouraging relaxation and awareness. You may alter your life by adopting healthy behaviors that encouraging productivity and well-being.

98. TAKING TIME TO RELAX AND RECHARGE, WHETHER THROUGH NAPPING OR DOING SOMETHING YOU ENJOY

Finding time to rest and recharge in today's fast-paced environment might be difficult. However, as part of a healthy lifestyle, it is essential to emphasize rest. Rest and recharge may assist in decreasing stress, improving mental health, and increasing general well-being.

Napping is one of the most efficient methods to relax and refresh. Napping has Numerous health advantages, including enhanced cognitive performance, greater alertness, and stress reduction. Several research studies show that sleeping regularly may reduce the risk of heart disease and other chronic conditions.

It is critical to keep naps brief and to the point. A 20-30-minute power nap may offer an immediate energy boost and enhance cognitive performance. Longer naps, on the other hand, may leave you sleepy and interrupt your sleep pattern. Furthermore, sleeping too late in the day may make it difficult to fall asleep at night.

Aside from sleeping, there are several additional methods to unwind and recover. Hobbies or activities you like, such as reading, art, or gardening, might be beneficial way to relax and decompress. Mindfulness or meditation may also be an effective approach to alleviate stress and quiet the mind.

It's vital to remember that relaxing does not always imply doing nothing. Physical activities like walking or performing yoga may also help you relax and recharge. Exercise has been proven to promote mental health and decrease stress, making it an important part of a healthy lifestyle.

It is critical to schedule time for self-care in addition to resting and indulging in hobbies and activities. Taking a warm bath, massage, or practicing proper sleep hygiene are all examples of self-care. Making self-care a priority helps decrease stress, improve mental health, and increase general well-being.

Making time to unwind and recharge is critical to living a healthy lifestyle. It is critical to emphasize relaxation via sleeping, hobbies and activities, or self-care. You may decrease stress, boost mental health, and increase general well-being.

99. MAKING TIME FOR SELF-CARE AND ACTIVITIES THAT SUPPORT YOUR WELL-BEING

Self-care is an essential component of total health and well-being. It entails taking deliberate measures to prioritize your mental, emotional, and physical well-being and scheduling activities to encourage self-love and happiness. Prioritizing self-care may result in various advantages, including lower stress, greater mood, enhanced productivity, and improved relationships.

A lack of time is one of the major barriers to self-care. Many believe they are too busy to put their health and well-being first. Self-care, on the other hand, is not a luxury; it is a requirement. It is important to arrange time in your calendar for activities that boost your well-being.

Making a list of things that make you happy and calm is one of the easiest methods to prioritize self-care. This might include reading a book, having a bubble bath, going for a nature walk, or doing yoga. Once you have created your list, attempt to include at least one of these activities in your daily routine.

Taking care of your physical health is another important part of self-care. This entails eating a well-balanced diet. Get adequate sleep and exercise regularly. A diet high in fruits, vegetables, whole grains, and lean meats will help fuel your body and provide you the energy you need to get through the day. Sleep is also important because it helps your body to rejuvenate and restore itself. Regular exercise may help you feel better, decrease stress, and enhance your health.

Prioritizing your mental and emotional well-being is equally critical. This may include mindfulness, meditation, or therapy. Taking time to focus on your thoughts and emotions may aid in the processing and managing of stress. It may also assist you in developing a more optimistic attitude toward life.

In addition to these solitary activities, it is critical to emphasize interpersonal interactions as part of self-care. A solid support network may assist in decreasing stress, boosting mood, and promoting general well-being. Contact loved ones regularly via phone, text message, or in-person visits.

To summarize, prioritizing self-care is critical for overall health and well-being. It entails taking deliberate measures to prioritize your mental, emotional, and physical well-being and scheduling activities to encourage self-love and happiness. By adding self-care into your daily routine, you may decrease stress, enhance mood, boost productivity, and establish stronger relationships. Remember that self-care is not a luxury; it is a must. Make time for yourself and put your health and well-being first.

100. PRACTICING GRATITUDE AND APPRECIATION FOR THE PRESENT MOMENT.

Gratitude and appreciation for the present moment are strong habits that may dramatically improve one's life. We may create a positive perspective and discover more meaning and purpose by focusing on the present and recognizing the wonderful things around us.

Gratitude is a mental attitude in which we recognize and appreciate the wonderful parts of our existence. It entails concentrating on the excellent things we have rather than what we lack or what has gone wrong. Gratitude practice has been demonstrated in studies to provide several advantages, including enhanced mental health, greater happiness, and improved relationships.

Keeping a gratitude notebook is one method to build thankfulness. This is writing down things you are thankful for daily, such as excellent health, supportive friends and family, or a gorgeous sunset. You may change your attention away from negative thoughts and emotions and build a more optimistic attitude by dwelling on the good parts of your life.

Another approach to demonstrate thankfulness is to convey thanks to the people in your life. This might be thanking a friend for their help or notifying a friend about your situation. Telling a family member how much you appreciate them, or even writing a letter of appreciation to a coworker who has helped you at work, is a kind gesture. You may deepen your connections and create a more pleasant, supportive environment around you by expressing thanks to others.

It is essential to enjoy the current moment in addition to growing thankfulness. This entails being present and immersed in your activity rather than continuously reflecting on the past or worrying about the future. You may feel more pleasure and contentment in your everyday life by concentrating on the now.

Mindfulness is one technique for appreciating the present moment. Mindfulness entails paying attention to the current moment without judgment. It may be developed via meditation, yoga, or just taking a few deep breaths and concentrating on your bodily sensations. Mindfulness allows you to become more aware of your thoughts and emotions and create more resilience and inner strength.

Engaging in things that offer pleasure and contentment is another approach to enjoying the present moment. This might be taking up a new activity, spending time with loved ones, or enjoying a gorgeous sunset or a good dinner. You may establish a stronger sense of purpose and meaning by planning activities that enjoy and satisfy you.

In conclusion, cultivating thankfulness and appreciation for the present moment are strong habits that have the potential to improve your life. By developing thankfulness, you may build a more positive view and enjoy higher pleasure, better mental health, and stronger relationships. You may feel more pleasure and contentment in your everyday life by enjoying the present moment and building a stronger sense of purpose and significance. By incorporating these habits into your daily routine, you can live a happier, healthier, and more satisfying life.

CONCLUSION

PUTTING IT ALL TOGETHER: YOUR ACTION PLAN

Achieving a healthy lifestyle might be difficult, but it is doable with the correct mentality, methods, and resources. We will offer you an action plan in this part to help you put all you have learned into practice.

Define Your Goals

It is critical to identify your goals before making changes to your lifestyle. What do you hope to accomplish? Do you want to reduce weight, get in shape, or feel better? Make your goals specific, measurable, and achievable by writing them down.

Make a Strategy

Create a strategy to assist you in reaching your goals once you have identified them. Begin by adopting tiny, manageable adjustments to your lifestyle, such as eating more fruits and vegetables, drinking more water, and going for a 10-minute walk every day. You may raise the complexity of your goals as you notice progress.

Build Healthy Habits

Building healthy habits is one of the cornerstones of living a healthy lifestyle. Begin by recognizing the bad habits holding you back, such as eating junk food or not getting enough sleep, and then replace them with healthy ones, such as eating more fruits and vegetables or going to bed earlier. Building healthy habits takes time and work, but they will become second nature once you do.

Stay Accountable

Maintaining accountability is critical to reaching your goals. Share your goals with someone you can rely on, such as a friend or family member, and ask them to keep you responsible. You may also employ technology, such as a fitness tracker or calorie monitoring software, to help you remain on track.

Seek Professional Assistance

Seek expert assistance if you are having difficulty meeting your goals. A licensed nutritionist or personal trainer can provide tailored advice and assistance to help you overcome any hurdles you may encounter.

In conclusion, healthy lifestyles require a mix of mentality, methods, and instruments. You may achieve your goals by setting your goals, making a strategy, developing healthy habits, keeping responsible, and obtaining expert help. You may alter your life and become the greatest version of yourself if you seek assistance when needed.

STAYING ACCOUNTABLE AND CONTINUING TO GROW

Accountability is one of the most important aspects of success in transforming your life with healthy habits. Holding oneself responsible entails accepting responsibility for your actions and being devoted to your goals. Making long-term adjustments to your habits and lifestyle may be difficult without responsibility.

Tracking your progress is an excellent approach to remaining accountable. This may be accomplished by writing, utilizing a fitness app, or simply discussing your success with a friend or family member. You may find areas where you are succeeding and places where you may need to improve by frequently assessing your progress.

Having a support system is also a crucial component of accountability. Surrounding oneself with people who have similar aims and ideals as you may be very motivating and encouraging. This may involve enrolling in a fitness class, joining a support group, or finding an exercise partner. You may keep one another responsible and celebrate each other's victories by forming a support system.

Along with responsibility, it is critical to keep learning and pushing yourself. It is easy to become stuck in a rut and grow comfortable with your routines, but this might stymie your growth and cause stagnation. You may continue to push yourself and progress physically and intellectually by establishing new goals and trying new things.

Changing up your exercises is one method to keep progressing. Incorporating new exercises or enrolling in a new fitness class helps keep your body challenged and avoid monotony. Learning new skills, such as preparing nutritious foods or practicing mindfulness, may broaden your knowledge and improve your general well-being.

Keeping responsible and growing is critical to altering your life with healthy behaviors. You may remain motivated and inspired to reach your goals by monitoring your progress, creating a support system, and pushing yourself to do new things. Remember to focus on your goals and enjoy your accomplishments along the road.